SUPER REMEDIES
That Can Change Your Life

....

EDWARD SHALTS, M.D.,D.HT.

SHALTSUMA

DISCLAIMER: *This book is intended as a reference volume only, not as a medical manual. The material here is designed to help you make informed decisions about your health. It is not intended as a substitute for any treatment that may have been prescribed by your doctor. The publisher and author of this book do not dispense medical advice or prescribe the use of any technique as a form of treatment for physical, mental, or emotional problems without the advice of a physician, either directly or indirectly. The intent of the publisher and author is only to offer information of a general nature to help you in your quest for emotional, physical, and spiritual well-being. In the event you use any of the information in the book for yourself, the publisher and author assume no responsibility for your actions.*

Copyright © 2024 by Edward Shalts

All rights reserved. No part of this publication may be reproduced, distributed, or transmitted in any form or by any means, including photocopying, recording, or other electronic or mechanical methods, without the prior written permission of the publisher, except in the case of brief quotations embodied in critical reviews and certain other noncommercial uses permitted by copyright law. For permission, contact the author via the website below.

Shaltsuma / Edward Shalts
Sarasota, Florida
Website: drshalts.com

Cover design by Gus Yoo
Editing and book production by Stephanie Gunning

Portions of this book were previously published in *Easy Homeopathy: The 7 Essential Remedies You Need for Common Illness and First Aid* and *The American Institute of Homeopathy Handbook for Parents: A Guide to Healthy Treatment for Everything from Colds and Allergies to ADHD, Obesity, and Depression.*

Super Remedies/Edward Shalts —1st edition

Library of Congress Control Number: 2024918625

ISBN 979-8-9901944-0-3 (paperback)
ISBN 979-8-9901944-1-0 (ebook)

To my grandson, Noah, with hope that he'll benefit from the information contained in this book. And to my daughters, Dora and Polina, and my partner and soul mate, Alina, with deep appreciation for being given a chance to meet these amazing human beings who continue to inspire me.

CONTENTS

Introduction   *1*

PART ONE
AN INTRODUCTION TO HOMEOPATHIC TREATMENT

1   Is It Healthy to Be Sick?   13
2   The Basic Principles of Homeopathy   27
3   How Homeopathic Remedies Are Made and Regulated   69
4   Myths, Controversy, and Confusion   99
5   Your Visit to the Homeopath   131
6   Instructions for Using Homeopathic Remedies   147

PART TWO
SUPER REMEDIES

7   Stramonium: Your Brother in Arms   153
8   Aconitum: Your Homeopathic Emergency Services Unit   167
9   Arnica: Your Homeopathic Surgeon   187
10   Belladonna: Your Homeopathic Pediatrician   215
11   Chamomilla: Your Homeopathic Babysitter   243
12   Gelsemium: Your Homeopathic Neurologist   267
13   Ignatia: Your Homeopathic Therapist   295

14 Nux Vomica: Your Homeopathic Gastroenterologist   321

15 Helpful Hints: Remedies for Common Ailments   371

16 Combination Remedies: An "Easy" Solution   401

Acknowledgments   *405*

End Notes   *407*

About the Author   *415*

If you are feeling sick, go to your medical doctor or to an urgent care center or the local emergency room.

Introduction

"The good physician treats the disease; the great physician treats the patient who has the disease."
—WILLIAM OSLER, M.D.

"The art of medicine consists of amusing the patient while nature cures the disease."
—VOLTAIRE

We were in a car, my mother and I, going to the cemetery to bury my father. As you can imagine, I knew my mother very well. I knew her better than anyone else in the world. I grew inside her. And after she gave me birth, I grew up with her—physically, emotionally, and mentally. She gave me everything that all humans want. She gave me *unconditional love.* I lived next to her and my father most of my life. My mother lived with my father for almost fifty years. And she also loved him unconditionally. She *really loved him.* Now he was gone.

My mother was a strong woman. Very strong. But she did not look strong on that sunny summer morning. She did not look strong at all. I said, "Ma, let me give you *Ignatia,* so you can make it to the funeral and stay OK. You look like you are about to die together with Shalts."

My father and I called each other Shalts. It was his idea. It made us feel special. He liked our last name. I like it, too. He called my mother simply Emma. He felt it was a strong name. As strong as she was.

I remember once trying to call my mother Emma, too, but she did not like it when I did. She said, "I am not an 'Emma' to you. I am your mama." So, we reached a consensus. I was allowed to call her Ma. To me "Ma" sounded like an abbreviation of "Mama Emma."

As I expected, my Mama Emma, the superwoman she was, said, "No, sonny, I am OK. I just have a horrible lump in my throat."

The next thing I knew, she was crying hysterically. We were fifteen to twenty minutes away from the cemetery. Again, I said, "Ma, you know you need it. Let me give you some *Ignatia*. Please!"

My mother was very much aware of homeopathy. She knew everything about me, including my love of homeopathy, and she knew the level of my medical skills. She had seen me in action on numerous occasions, prescribing remedies, and had witnessed homeopathy do miracles for her, my father, and my children. On this occasion, she accepted one dose of *Ignatia amara 30C.*

By the time we arrived at the cemetery, she felt calm. There was no lump in her throat anymore and she was able to go through the entire process of the burial without falling apart. Yes, she cried when the coffin was lowered into the grave, but there was no hysteria. Like her, I cried when I started saying the last words over my father's grave.

My mother continued to do well on the way home and during the meal that followed the ceremony. She cried again, of course, but did not feel distraught. My mother took another dose of *Ignatia* that night, and took a few more doses during the following week. She never felt overcome with grief again.

There you have it. My mother received the main homeopathic remedy for grief and a broken heart: *Ignatia amara.* Homeopaths simply call it *Ignatia.*

One of my recent patients agreed to provide a testimony for this book under her real name. Here it is.

> *Hello! My name is Megan Andrews. I am sharing with you the tremendous impact homeopathy has had on my life. Prior to*

meeting Dr. Shalts, I was not even the slightest bit aware of what homeopathy was. Shortly after learning about homeopathy and its benefits, he offered to sit down and consult me about a remedy for the symptoms I was having. After years of doctor appointments and tests with no answers to what was going on, I was skeptical of another consultation. The health issues I was experiencing were most definitely impacting my daily life, making me anxious to leave my house on certain days.

I'd had my gallbladder removed about a year before I started the homeopathic remedy. And even though having it removed helped me with the gallbladder attacks I was experiencing I was still struggling with certain aftereffects.

The consultation process with Dr. Shalts went extremely smoothly; after consulting with me a few times, he had chosen a remedy that he thought would help. Within the first few days of taking this remedy, I started to notice positive changes. My appetite, which usually wasn't present other than very late at night, was starting to come back. I began eating normally throughout the day and was able to stop snacking at inappropriate times of night. My stomach felt a lot better and I was able to tolerate foods I couldn't beforehand. The cramps I'd been getting disappeared. The aftereffects of having my gallbladder taken out were drastically improving. Overall, I felt like I had more energy—I wasn't nearly as sluggish as before. Unlike with pharmaceutical medicines that I've taken before, I did not experience any negative side effects.

Many times, I've heard an argument that I, as well as my fellow homeopaths, affect patients with my personality. The complaint is that we kind of hypnotize them, so that the "empty" sugar pill I give them works as a powerful placebo. Of course, I could remind these naive skeptics that the homeopathic remedies I prescribe for my patients are bought at a store or online, and then taken by those patients at random times. Or I could dedicate a whole chapter or a whole book to presenting detailed evidence countering the idea of a "sugar pill" or placebo (and things like that have been written before by numerous authors).

If you who want to look into these issues at a different level, I recommend starting from reading an article I cowrote with the esteemed integrative physician Woodson Merrell, M.D., simply entitled "Homeopathy," published in *Medical Clinics of North America*, vol. 86, no. 1 (January 2002): pages 47–62.

I think I should also tell you the story of a ferret who weaseled his way out of death.

In 1997, I met an artist who came to me as a patient for various problems. We developed a pretty good rapport and at the end of the interview when I asked her whether there is anything else I could help her with, the artist told me: "I have a ferret. His name is Rat-Rat because this is the noise he makes all the time. I've had him for so many years. He is such a weasel! I love him so much! But he is dying now.

"Maybe it is OK for him to die, as he is kind of old, but he seems to be in awful pain, and he stopped eating and has such terrible diarrhea. He's lost so much weight. I heard that homeopathy could help people to die peacefully. Is there anything in homeopathy to help an animal to die in a decent way?"

I said: "Well, we have this remedy called *Arsenicum album*. It is known to help people in terminal stages of their life to die painlessly and in peace. It also helps for diarrhea. Maybe Rat-Rat will benefit from it."

She said: "OK. We've got nothing to lose. He is dying anyway."

I informed her that *Arsenicum album* 30C would probably be easy for her to find in her local health food store.

We met again in a month for her follow-up. At the end of our discussion about her own health improvements, the artist said, "By the way, Rat-Rat weaseled his way out of death. After I gave him the remedy, his diarrhea stopped. Now, he is not in pain and he is eating. He is also fat again!" Every time we met for the next couple of years, the artist gave me a positive report about the ferret.

Here is a real miracle that we can attribute to homeopathy, even considering that we had to deal with a weasel.

I believe that my patient's ferret simply had a case of severe diarrhea that was helped by *Arsenicum,* which is one of the main remedies any of us would take for diarrhea and food poisoning. I've seen many other cases when the only thing that any remedy, homeopathic or allopathic could do, even in the best-case scenario, was to ease the suffering of a dying person or an animal.

A few years later I had an opportunity to meet with the family of a prominent fashion photographer. They had a few children with various health issues, so I made a home visit to see them in their natural environment. At the end of the visit, the photographer offered me a cup of tea. We were sitting in the kitchen which had a tile floor. It was summertime. They had a few dogs. One was lying on the cold floor on her left side. I asked the owner why this dog was lying on the tiles. She responded: " I don't know. But ever since Daisy developed a horrible ear infection, she's been doing this. I don't think homeopathy would work for an animal, otherwise you'd have another patient."

When I responded that I didn't specialize in the treatment of animals, but there are veterinarian homeopaths who do, she was surprised. (Maybe you are surprised too.) She asked, "Do you think you could try anyway?"

By that time I already knew a few important things. The dog:

1. Had an ear infection.

2. Felt better from exposure to a cold temperature. She herself had chosen to lay on the cool tile floor.)
3. Was lying on her left side.

To make sure I was not mistaken about the best remedy to give the dog, I asked which side the ear infection was on. The owner responded, "On the left."

I asked what else the owner noticed about the dog. Her response confirmed my thoughts about a particular remedy. She said, "Daisy has been spending all her time on my lap. She has never been so affectionate before. Maybe it's from pain."

To me, an experienced homeopath (I'm making this point to discourage you from self-prescribing based on this story), the choice of remedy was clear. I said to the dog's owner: "If it was my child, I'd give her *Pulsatilla* in concentration 30C."

As I learned a few days later, the dog got much better after a few doses of the remedy. This case illustrates an important feature of homeopathy. The choice of remedy is based on the individual characteristics of the person being treated, including facts like their emotional state and even such things as the location of their symptoms. Homeopathy is truly holistic, as it treats a whole person, not just a single symptom at a time.

By now, I suspect that you may be asking yourself the question: "If even fifty percent of what this guy's telling me is true, how come homeopathy hasn't taken over the world?!"

A VERY reasonable question!

The simple answer to it is that homeopathy does not fit into the simplistic approach to health which has been adopted by modern western society.

Homeopathy dominated the medical scene of the western world, including the scene in the United States, until the early 1920s. By that time the industrial revolution had taken over the world and the huge masses of people who moved into cities were demanding medical services that could address their issues quickly in a uniform fashion. Homeopaths could not satisfy these criteria as homeopathic prescription is highly individualized and, with a few remarkable exceptions that are described in this book, one remedy does not fit all the cases most of the time. On the other hand, allopathic medicine (aka conventional medicine) had by this point started developing effective antibacterial medications and surgery with anesthesia had made advances too.

Furthermore, cocky homeopathic leadership, which was used to build enormous success for homeopathic practitioners from the late 1880s through the early 1900s, refused to adapt the curriculum of homeopathic schools to new, stricter educational standards established by the U.S. government. The game was over. The success of conventional medicine in treating the wounded during World War I and, later World War II, combined with the earlier discoveries of vaccination and antibiotics, served the final blow to homeopathy. In the United States, homeopathy went underground, while in most European countries it has remained one of the widely accepted methods of treatment.

A significantly more detailed account of this process is described in the book *Divided Legacy,* written by Harris Coulter.

What is important to us is that homeopathy is still alive and can be super helpful in many acute situations. It can be a game changer in treating chronic illnesses. You can get more information about finding qualified providers to consult from the American Institute of Homeopathy (AIH) and the National Center for Homeopathy (NCH).

It is actually a miracle that homeopathy still exists in the United States, given the history of its downfall. The only explanation for this phenomenon I have is that homeopathy remains amazingly efficient when master practitioners practice it. Therefore, it is difficult to discount completely.

I have to say that homeopathic organizations remain feisty and have fought many innovations important for public health, including mass vaccinations. This has been a great disadvantage to homeopathy as a movement.

As you can see, the lack of acceptance of homeopathy by conventional medicine, and consequently by the majority of the general population, has deep roots, and those for or against homeopathy have played roles in making things difficult.

Some countries are more fortunate when it comes to homeopathy. India, for example, has over 200,000 practicing homeopathic medical doctors. Their presentations at international conferences are simply amazing. Homeopathy is also rapidly developing where it used to be unknown. For example, in Turkey.

The argument that homeopathy is only popular in "third-world" nations because it is cheap and many people in these countries cannot afford to purchase conventional medications is unfair and inaccurate, as the economies of these countries are developing rapidly. India just landed a rocket on the moon and Turkey is a well-developed industrial country.

Clinically, hundreds of thousands of cured cases have been documented in the vast homeopathic literature and presented at numerous homeopathic conferences around the world. Homeopathy has been a life-changing experience for hundreds of thousands of children. Acute situations such as croup, for example, for which there is no effective conventional treatment, can be resolved literally in minutes by homeopathic treatment.

Common sense as well as history advise that the best way to find out whether homeopathy is an effective method of treatment or a fake is to try it in simple, nonthreatening situations. You can always take a homeopathic remedy on your way to urgent care or the emergency room.

Opponents of homeopathy say it is just an "empty" sugar pill. So there can be no negative effects, right? You've got nothing to lose, but potentially, you might gain rapid improvement and a cure of a medical problem.

Another, rather obvious question you might have is "Why does the book talk so much about children?"

The answer is simple. The bodies and minds of children have enormous plasticity. They are constantly growing and developing. And we want to help them the best we can to grow strong, healthy, and smart. In order to achieve these goals in an optimal way, we need to allow our children's bodies and minds to learn how to best interact with the environment they were born into using their innate capacity to adapt and to develop.

From this point of view, allowing a child to get over a common cold without utilization of powerful antibiotics or hormones is a good idea. Homeopathy can often do better with routine health-care issues than medication. When used appropriately, homeopathy can cure common colds, acute digestive issues, and acute allergic reactions literally in minutes. I could not even tell how many hundreds of thousands of children with teething problems have been helped. (And if you ever had to experience long, sleepless nights watching your child suffering, screaming, and being unable to sleep because of teething pain, you know the urgency of addressing this issue.) An experienced homeopath may be able to help a child to overcome allergies, chronic asthma, frequent ear infections, eczema, chronic indigestion, and even severe nightmares.

Allowing our children to overcome health issues quickly without utilizing powerful drugs is a life-changing proposition—especially considering that nowadays we have access to conventional doctors, emergency rooms, and powerful drugs and can always bring our children to a medical doctor or ER should natural treatment fail.

Just to give a simple example, is there anything one can do if stung by a bee and developing a horrible swelling before giving a powerful drug? The answer is yes, take a homeopathic remedy *Apis mellifica* 30C on your way to the nearest ER. In the best-case scenario, the swelling will be gone by the time you arrive. In the worst-case scenario, the swelling will continue and you or your child will be in the ER just in time to receive qualified medical treatment. No harm will be done.

I want to emphasize that this book is not an attempt to diminish the important role of contemporary medicine in improving your quality of life and saving lives every day. My intention is to provide you with comprehensive information about several very effective alternatives, which I am calling *super remedies,* that may come in handy for you, your family (especially your children), and your friends and neighbors. There is nothing else available from other types of medicine that compares to super remedies when it comes to the treatment of many conditions.

I am a medical doctor as well as a homeopathic physician, and I have spent over forty years of my life witnessing the literal miracles produced by homeopathy first hand. I wrote two books on homeopathy that were published about twenty years ago, but both of those older books are basically sold out now, and the world has changed quite a bit, so I decided to publish this new book. It combines information on homeopathy that remains accurate and proven by years of practice with additional material that should be helpful to people who suffer from post-trauma and stress (this probably describes most of us).

PART ONE

AN INTRODUCTION TO HOMEOPATHIC TREATMENT

CHAPTER ONE

Is It Healthy to Be Sick?

"Do not swat the fly on your friend's head with a hatchet."
—CONFUCIUS

You and your family deserve to have access to the best health care available—care that is noninvasive, produces no negative side effects, and doesn't cost an arm and a leg in the bargain. That's why *Super Remedies* exists. The eight primary homeopathic remedies in this book, and their seventy-nine secondary counterparts, form the basis of a first-aid protocol that you can rapidly learn to use to effectively complement your conventional medical care. When they are appropriately applied, these homeopathic remedies can swiftly relieve discomfort so you and your loved ones may get on with the important daily matters of living. After all, good health is the foundation of everything we do in our lives.

You picked up this book because you're interested in learning more about homeopathy, an intervention that helps the body naturally respond better to whatever physical, emotional, and mental challenges it faces. *Super Remedies* covers sudden, short-term problems. Homeopathy has been proven effective in the treatment of acute ailments, such as the common cold, diarrhea, and earache, as well as in the treatment of chronic diseases, such as allergies and panic disorder.

Before you will be ready to put homeopathy to practical use, there are a few important concepts you need to understand, starting with the nature of homeopathic remedies and how they can serve you. We will discuss these concepts in this chapter.

What Are Homeopathic Remedies?

Homeopathy is a medical specialty that uses diluted natural substances, known as *remedies,* to stimulate the body's innate capacity for healing. These remedies have been both diluted and shaken multiple times in order to give them potency. Oddly, the more times remedies are diluted and shaken—in other words, the less concentrated they are—the stronger they become. And substances that are diluted *without* being shaken do not produce the same healing effects in those who consume them as the ones that have been shaken. No one knows exactly why this is true, even though it is what the clinical and laboratory research has confirmed.

Why do we use diluted substances to make homeopathic remedies? According to the principle that "like cures like," which is the foundation of homeopathy, any substance that causes a combination of symptoms in a healthy, sensitive individual can cure similar symptoms in the sick. Essentially, homeopathy gives us a nonharmful way to sample a "poison." Remedies are so thoroughly diluted that we can barely detect the raw material.

Homeopathy was discovered by a German physician, chemist, and pharmacologist named Samuel Hahnemann over two hundred years ago. Since then, homeopathic remedies have proven enormously successful in providing individualized help and highly effective cures for many illnesses without causing any side effects or complications. They are also easy to use, because each remedy is prescribed only to cure a unique constellation of symptoms—a picture, if you will. When the patient and the remedy share an identical picture, you give it. If they don't, you make a different choice. Choosing a remedy for an acute condition is relatively straightforward because acute conditions tend to present clear, easy-to-see symptoms.

Perhaps the most difficult concept to grasp about homeopathy, albeit the one that makes it so incredibly powerful, is that at any given moment there is only one special remedy a person would benefit from taking. Whenever you can identify this correct remedy, it initiates a cascade of healing throughout the recipient's entire integrated being. A single remedy can improve that person's physical, emotional, and mental well-being.

A Few of the Reasons That Homeopathy Is More Important Today Than Ever Before

After we are born, our bodies need training in order to learn what to do and then, later, to upgrade to proficiency. Just think about it. It takes infants a while to learn how to walk without falling down and to speak in full sentences. Developing these skills involves frequent stimulation from their parents and other adults. Isolated infants and toddlers fail to acquire intellectual skills that are even close to those of normal toddlers. Similarly, the immune system needs training. In order to remain healthy, it must be able to differentiate between life forms that are its "friends" and its "enemies." Children who've been given the chance to encounter different germs are more proficient at averting disease.

A backyard in the country and a sandbox in the city are excellent training grounds for the immune system. In these environments, children touch different objects, including the soil, plants, worms, other children, and so forth, giving them exposure to various microbes—bacteria and viruses (aka "bugs"). The immune system fights back, often winning right away and growing stronger as a result. Other times an infection occurs. The immune system learns from that experience, too. A fever speeds up the production of immune cells and creates an unfriendly environment in the body for the bugs. A bunch of other symptoms also develop that indicate the body is undergoing a healing process. If sick children are kept home for a few days, so the immune system has enough time and acceptable conditions to get over the aggression, it becomes smarter, more capable.

A cold? Yes! Bring it on! Time to have a training fight! That's the attitude I'd like to see more parents adopt. But this rarely occurs anymore. Nowadays, there's an active exchange of viruses between exhausted schoolchildren who were sent to class by parents after receiving doses of fever medication and decongestants. This exchange is unrestricted by natural defense mechanisms. Rather than fighting bugs naturally, most kids don't get the rest they need and aren't allowed to experience the healing mechanisms of their symptoms. Powerful medications (often unnecessary) prevent them from having a fever to speed up the immune response and having nasal discharges that flush their bodies out. If modern families reversed the cultural tendency to suppress symptoms and let children be a little sick from time to time, we would be a much healthier society.

Does this advice seem primitive to you? Perhaps. But there's scientific evidence that it is reliable advice. As it turns out, many children in developing countries still live much as children in the industrialized nations did in the 1950s. Interestingly, although these children often suffer from diseases related to poverty and poor hygiene, they have significantly fewer chronic illnesses like allergies. In simple terms, allergic reactions are the result of an uneducated immune system that doesn't know what to do. By overreacting to natural substances, like pollen, that normally wouldn't be perceived as an "enemy" the immune system turns against the body it's supposed to protect.

At the top of the chapter, I cited a quote from Confucius, "Do not swat a fly on your friend's head with a hatchet." You're probably wondering: *What's the big deal? That's so obvious!* Well, not really. You see, in western medicine we typically take a shock-and-awe approach to disease, with an emphasis on wiping out symptoms rather than viewing symptoms as signs of healing process.

Parents blame physicians for overprescribing medications. Physicians respond that frequently they are driven by a wish of parents to do everything possible to "protect" children from infections and complications. The same situation it true for adults. I can't even begin to tell you how often patients walk into my office and say, "Doctor, I need an antidepressant!" or "Doc, I am studying for a difficult test. Give me a prescription for a stimulant." (They will actually name a drug they saw advertised.)

Who is in the right and who is in the wrong here? As always, the answer rests right smack in the middle. We, parents and doctors alike, grew up in a culture of fear, constantly feeling as if we are in a medical emergency. Pain? Take painkillers! Fever? Suppress it! Where did this attitude come from? Obviously, there are many possible explanations. The most obvious is the history of medicine in the twentieth century.

Proprietary medications—drugs that are patented and earn companies revenue—first appeared on the market after successful trials that took place during World War I. Being able to respond immediate to potentially disabling problems was critical to the success of the army. Wound—pain—immediate removal of pain and suffering. "Stitch 'em up, and send 'em back to the battlefield." Another major development was the Industrial Revolution. Businesses adopted a militaristic sense of urgency. Thousands of people had to get to work every day. Like foot soldiers, they had to get better immediately—*no matter what*. Missing work, even to rest and support the body's functions, was seen as a disaster to be prevented by heroic measures.

A false feeling of omnipotence was also born in western culture as a result of our great technological advances. We believed that the human body was similar to a machine and interventions would keep it running more efficiently. These two concepts—urgent care and the sense that we knew almost everything—drove medicine and our mentality for over a century. Certainly, it was a self-fulfilling prophecy. Vaccinations eliminated deadly infections, sophisticated anesthesia and painkillers diminished pain, antibiotics were killing germs, and powerful psychotropic medications seemed to make psychiatric patients so much better. We bought into it.

Today, people go on the internet to do research so they can ask the right questions of their doctors. The impulse is pure, and there's also an inherent watchfulness. Doctors are aware of third parties, including lawyers, insurance companies, bureaucrats, and the media, who are looking over their shoulders all the time to ensure they'll do what is "safe" and "correct." The trouble is that society often considers it safest to apply heroic measures to simple situations. We use drugs to decrease minor fevers. We turn to major antibiotics every time a person has a head cold. We use antidepressants to cope with normal grief or situational anxiety. Not only do doctors prescribe drugs for acute care, but patients also ask for these drugs by name (they've seen them advertised) because they live in a state of constant fear of a disaster that might possibly happen if... There's a sense that nature must be controlled and overcome. There's a lack of faith in the wisdom of the body.

Somehow I don't think you are surprised by this logic. You are probably reading this book partly because you are aware that new, equally disturbing health problems have replaced the ones we "removed." Epidemics of acute infectious diseases, like measles and polio, have been replaced by epidemics of chronic illnesses, such as asthma, cancer, irritable bowel syndrome, and even obesity. We are facing antibiotic-resistant infections for which doctors still recommend the use of powerful antibiotics.

A Better Approach

As a society, we managed to ignore the big picture for more than a century. Now we are learning that we were prodding a sophisticated, gentle device called a *human being* with coarse, unsophisticated tools. Although these tools brought us some temporary relief, in fact they ended up causing us more complex, systemic health problems.

Think back to the Confucius quote at the beginning of the chapter. Haven't we been swatting at flies with a hatchet? Actually, I'd rather use the analogy of a sledgehammer. We typically beat our symptoms with a sledgehammer of powerful medications. As symptoms get suppressed, more complicated, deeper-seated problems come out.

Drugs *affect* entire human beings. While their intended effects suppress the symptoms of disease or kill the intruders, their many other unintended consequences—*side effects*—can hurt us. We often indirectly cause our bodies damage by jumping into the middle of the fight between the powerful defense forces given to us by Mother Nature (the immune system is only one of them) and an intruder.

What steps, if any, can we take today to undo the potential harm, as well as the clear and present harm, of overmedicating ourselves? First, we have to stop panicking. It is important to consider our methods of healthcare reasonably. We need to understand when we truly need to intervene with drugs, surgery, and so on. Secondly, the rest of the time we can successfully call upon the miracle of homeopathy, a method of healthcare that gives us the freedom to eliminate illness using our own nature-given devices.

The Four Levels of Health

How can you and your family begin to achieve optimal health? Developing a reasonable and trustworthy healthcare strategy that blends conventional medicine and homeopathy becomes much easier if you understand the four possible levels of health.[1]

Level 1 Health

In *The Jungle Book,* Rudyard Kipling tells the story of a boy living in harmony with nature: "Now you must be content to . . . guess at all the wonderful life that Mowgli led among the wolves . . . He grew up with the cubs . . . and Father Wolf taught him his business, and the meaning of things in the jungle . . . When he was not learning he sat out in the sun and slept, and ate, and went to sleep again; when he felt dirty or hot he swam in the forest pools; and when he wanted honey . . . he climbed up for it . . . And he grew and grew strong as a boy must grow, who does not know that he is learning any lessons."[2]

A city dweller myself, I am far from suggesting that everyone has to live with the wolves in order to be healthy. The important point in my interpretation of the story is that Mowgli grew up strong because he was in constant contact with nature. His body learned quickly what was a "friend" or an "enemy." Although Kipling wasn't specifically writing about it, Mowgli's body would have had no confusion, no allergic reactions. The only help available to the child was good advice from Father Wolf and a few other animals. His body would have been perfectly able to deal with the adversities of daily life. If Mowgli had a cut, he would have had to deal with it. Maybe Baloo, the brown bear, would offer him some herbs to speed up the healing. If he had a cold, he would have had to deal with it. Maybe Bagheera, the black panther, would bring him some honey to speed his recovery.

We rarely see this level of health in city dwellers. But I can easily imagine a shepherd from the Alps or a cowboy possessing a strong immune system and having no health problems, even in old age. These people represent the first level of health. Strong and resilient, they are fully capable of dealing with seasonal infections and minor traumas without needing constant support from antibiotics and painkillers. They haven't been exposed to the devastating attacks of noise, chemical pollution, and emotional strain so readily provided by our civilization. We all strive to be at this level of health, but few who live in the industrial world are.

All the supplements and vitamins we take, and all the dieting and exercise to which we subject ourselves have one ultimate goal: to make us healthy and achieve the magical level of wellness. People with Level 1 health recover completely from acute problems. They have chronic diseases neither of the body nor of the mind. If they develop any difficulties during recovery, a single dose of a homeopathic remedy brings them right back to where they were before.

When people grow up surrounded by nature and then become city dwellers, their ability to resist illness remains strong for many years despite encountering the adversities and stresses of the industrialized world. Why? Because their major defense systems formed under ideal conditions. Their bodies learn how to resist disease by themselves, without the interference of external agents or pollutants, and also without the unnecessary suppression of symptoms by powerful drugs.

Prior to the introduction in daily life of chemical and psychological pollutants, the majority of the population that survived different disease epidemics most likely was at Level 1 of health. For a few generations after industrialization, humans were able to resist the negative impact of manmade pollutants, but a consistent and powerful widespread assault ultimately brought about a collective decrease in our resistance. We are rapidly moving down the ladder of health.

Let's see what's awaiting us, dwellers in the so-called civilized world of the twenty-first century at the second level of health.

Level 2 Health

The classic short story "Hygeia at the Solito" by O. Henry is one of my favorites, as it so clearly illustrates how people with Level 2 health are capable of shifting to Level 1. In the tale, "Cricket" McGuire, described as an "ex-feather-weight prizefighter, tout, jockey, follower of the 'ponies,' all-round sport, and manipulator of the gumballs and walnut shells," has been diagnosed with tuberculosis and given an estimated six months to live. Then, altruistic cattleman Curtis Raidler rescues him by speeding him off to his ranch. Raidler is the picture of robust health and vitality, physically and emotionally.[3]

"Thus was instituted the reign of terror at the Solito Ranch," according to Henry. McGuire, a truly heinous individual, sits in his room with the windows closed smoking cigarettes and trying to figure out a way to scam everyone around him. He's ornery and egotistical, and complains nonstop. This goes on for two months, during which time he doesn't improve. Yes, he's got lung disease, but he's also strong and wiry.

If it weren't for his chronic cough, you might believe he was a fairly healthy, if unpleasant, individual.

Raidler offers the man some Level 1 healthcare advice. "Try more air, son.... The ground, and the air next to it—them's the things to cure you.... Close to the ground—that's where the medicine in the air stays. Try a little hossback riding now." When this counsel is rejected, Raidler begins to be suspicious. One evening, he asks a dinner guest—a physician—to examine McGuire.

Another thing I like about this story is that a major plot twist comes from a doctor making a mistake. "In ten minutes the doctor came briskly out. 'Your man,' he said promptly, 'is as sound as a new dollar.... I advise you to set him digging post-holes or breaking mustangs.'" Of course, he has examined the wrong man.

Raidler takes his advice. "'Take this man,' said Raidler to Ross Hargis, 'and put him to work. Make him work hard, sleep hard, and eat hard.'" From obstinacy McGuire doesn't correct their illusion and just goes along. The rancher goes off to take care of family business in another state and doesn't return for two months, at which point he comes home, discovers the doctor's error, and is persuaded that McGuire must be dead. He races out to the encampment where he learns that McGuire is thriving. The doctor's mistake was his salvation. Fresh air, exercise, and simple food were what he needed.

Of course, I would not go so far as to suggest treating tuberculosis with exercise in the prairies. But, as you can see from the story, people who have Level 2 health are normally healthy people—the primary readership of this book! Typically, they are overworked, stressed, and victims of pollution. Although the body fights against viruses, it wins in the long-term, not immediately.

There's an old joke that applies to this group. A common cold goes away in fourteen days with treatment and in two weeks without treatment. But these odds can be improved. Level 2 people can shift to Level 1 with the use of homeopathy, because it stimulates self-healing and restoration of powerful defenses.

Level 3 Health

Level 3 health describes chronically ill people who have one or more serious illnesses, such as ongoing asthma and chronic ulcers. Where Level 1 people might get colds once or twice a year and Level 2 people might get colds several times a year, Level 3 people rarely get colds because their defenses are overstimulated and always operating on "high alert." It's like having a firewall up on your computer—anything that enters the system just gets burned up.

Whereas at Level 2 the situation is not life threatening, at Level 3 it has the potential to be. The goal of homeopathic treatment, which must be provided by trained professionals once you're dealing with this category of ill health, is to help people to advance to Level 2. If they develop an acute problem, it creates a window of opportunity to improve their overall level of health, as it reveals new symptoms.

At the beginning of the chapter, when we were discussing homeopathic remedies, I explained that there is only one perfect remedy for each person at a given time. The process of homeopathy is always to identify the special remedy that matches an individual's unique picture of symptoms. As you read chapters seven through sixteen, you'll find descriptions of the leading indicators for the different homeopathic remedies. Having extra symptoms to work on matching in Level 3 cases can help us prescribe a breakthrough remedy.

Level 4 Health

Terminally ill people fall into the Level 4 category. As their defenses are completely exhausted, the body succumbs to the illness. The best we can do for them is offer palliation. This group of people requires sophisticated, complicated treatment, which is far beyond the scope of this book.

The Goal of Homeopathy

The primary focus of this book is the treatment of acute ailments, which may be handled differently by people at the different levels of health. How so? And to what purpose?

Healthy people can sustain significant amounts of emotional and environmental stress, including viruses and bacteria. After a short and efficient struggle, which may produce a high fever and other temporarily debilitating symptoms, a healthy person (Level 1) eliminates the illness completely and returns to perfect health. They rarely need help to feel better. Such a person may decide to take it easy for a couple of days, or can take one dose of a homeopathic remedy, and will rapidly recover. This applies to healthy adults, infants, and children.

Most of us, however, live on the generally OK, second level of health (Level 2). We are striving to move up by improving our resilience. Effective homeopathic self-care can help us to achieve this goal both by treating our illnesses and by helping us to avoid the unwanted complications of suppressive conventional drug treatment.

People with serious chronic illnesses (Level 3) and those who have so far been unable to find a homeopathic solution for acute problems will benefit from professional homeopathic help and can gradually move to Level 2 and even Level 1 of health.

Now that you have a clearer understanding of the four levels of health, you are ready to learn the basic rules of homeopathy. Which remedy needs to be taken and which type of medical intervention needs to be sought both depend on the particular situation in which a particular person finds him or herself at the moment. The levels of health are just a simple tool to help you begin to assess your needs and set realistic expectations.

CHAPTER TWO

The Basic Principles of Homeopathy

"The privilege of a lifetime is being who you are."
—JOSEPH CAMPBELL

Without a doubt, this is the most important chapter in this book. In it, you'll learn what homeopathy is and how it differs from conventional, or *allopathic,* medicine. If you're a parent, I'd wager you're probably just looking to learn about a few homeopathic remedies so you can help your children, and I promise that you'll find such information in these pages. You're also likely also interested in addressing common complaints that you yourself are experiencing. Yet homeopathy differs enormously from conventional medicine and give accomplish bigger things. Therefore, before you can set out on course of homeopathic healing, you need to understand a few significant details. Otherwise, you may be as astonished and disbelieving as Tim's parents were when they saw the results their kid got.

As happens frequently in my homeopathic practice, I saw Tim after his parents had already tried every single conventional approach offered to them by dermatologists. Tim was thirteen and he had an awful case of eczema. Lesions had spread all over his body, most looking like various stages of poison ivy, and they were, as Tim put it, "very ugly." The itching was enormous. Luckily, he only had a few marks on his face.

Tim and his parents felt devastated. This good-looking, intelligent boy couldn't socialize, as he was afraid that other kids would make fun of him. He avoided going to the beach, swimming in the pool, or playing sports. After all, what if another student saw his embarrassing lesions while he was changing in the locker room? His parents were also concerned that the eczema wouldn't get better no matter what they did. They'd heard from dermatologists that kids usually "outgrow" eczema. But it hadn't happened so far.

As far as homeopathy is concerned, the severity of skin lesions doesn't matter as long as the patient is otherwise healthy. In our initial consultation, I determined that Tim was. I therefore knew I simply had to find the correct remedy with which to treat him. One dose of that exact remedy would probably take care of everything. Of course, this was easy for me to say. The parents told me honestly that if not for the utter failure of conventional treatments, including steroids, they would never have considered bringing their son to a homeopath. In the end, they only came because a mutual friend recommended me as trustworthy.

After taking a look at Tim's lesions, I conducted a full homeopathic interview. The questions I asked were seemingly strange. I was mostly interested in what made his rash feel better or worse, and in what made Tim different from other people. I wanted to know his eating and sleeping habits, and about his relationship with the weather, animals, and people. I needed to understand what made this particular child with eczema different from everyone else with the same diagnosis. In addition, I needed to match the set of symptoms that Tim was then exhibiting with the set of symptoms that had been triggered in healthy volunteers by a homeopathic substance during initial research conducted to understand its curative properties. That's how a homeopath carefully picks a remedy.

After about an hour and a half of conversation and evaluation, I made a decision. I gave Tim a 200C dose of a homeopathic remedy called *Rhus toxicodendron*. He dissolved the sugary pellet under his tongue and told me he liked its sweetness. I explained to his parents that I'd given him a preparation of poison ivy that had been diluted 10^{400} times. Tim's father was a chemist. He said, "That's crazy. Nothing diluted this much can work." Not only that, but he was also surprised I wanted Tim to take a pill only once. Both parents seemed disappointed that there was nothing else I was willing to offer. Nevertheless, they didn't have a choice.

I asked Tim's parents to wait six to eight weeks and then come in again for a follow-up appointment. Two months later, they brought Tim back. The rash was gone! Tim was so happy that he'd decided to become a homeopath when he grew up. They reported that about five days after taking the *Rhus,* Tim complained of an increased rash and itching. But a few days later, the itching subsided and the lesions started to disappear. The skin on the upper parts of his body healed first, and then the rash completely went away.

Interestingly, not all cases of eczema would have responded to *Rhus*. Truth be told, I've successfully prescribed many other remedies for the same skin condition. In homeopathy, we treat the individual patient rather than aiming to suppress the symptoms of a disease. Like Tim, his parents were thrilled with the results of homeopathy. But they still wondered if we should give Tim more of the remedy, just to make sure he would be fine in the future. I explained to them that "more" wasn't necessary, or even useful. He was cured.

What Is Homeopathy?

Homeopathy is a medical approach that's defined by the principle of similars: "Like cures like." Its practitioners use small quantities of highly diluted substances that in larger quantities would provoke the same symptoms they intend to cure. In the case of Tim, for instance, we employed heavily diluted poison ivy to heal an itchy skin rash. The idea is to give the body's own healing process a tiny boost. All forms of medicine that don't follow this principle are considered *allopathy*. In Latin, *allo* means "other" or "different," whereas *homo/homeo* means "same" or "similar." The medical suffix *pathy* comes from the root word *pathos,* meaning "suffering" or "disease." Samuel Hahnemann coined the names for both medical approaches.

In homeopathy, we appreciate symptoms as being the language in which the body speaks to us. They show us that the body is struggling to externalize the potential damage that a deep-seated illness could do at the body's core. If we're seeing various external symptoms, we can be fairly certain that deep damage hasn't been done yet. If these stop, we can assume that either the individual is cured or the illness has reached deeper to the core level.

In allopathy, symptoms are viewed as *being* an illness, rather than signs of the body's attempt to heal, which is why conventional doctors believe they must be suppressed. By contrast, homeopathy views the body's expression of symptoms as a healthy restorative mechanism. For this reason, homeopaths treat a patient's set of symptoms with remedies that would cause a similar set of symptoms if taken in sufficient quantity by a healthy person. Like cures like.

The Principle of Similars

Samuel Hahnemann was an extraordinarily intelligent and multitalented man. Born April 10, 1755, into the family of a poor German porcelain painter, he had to work from a young age. At twelve, he was already tutoring Greek. Later on he became a prolific writer, translator, doctor, chemist, and pharmacologist. Once he presented a thesis in Latin at the University of Leipzig. During this presentation, Hahnemann apparently quoted sources in eight original languages, including Hebrew and Arabic.

A tragic misconception about homeopathy is that it has no scientific basis. This statement couldn't be further from the truth. As you read on, I'm sure you'll appreciate how much Hahnemann has done for modern biomedical science. He introduced many groundbreaking ideas into medical practice. Hahnemann discovered homeopathy at age thirty-five by conducting a series of experiments on himself. In the process, he invented reliable research methods. Prior to that, he was already deeply involved with nutrition and noninvasive healing. We're talking about the 1700s here! Clearly a man way ahead of his time, without any doubt, Hahnemann deserves recognition as being the father of modern scientifically based medicine, both homeopathic and conventional.

Hahnemann's discovery of homeopathy began when he was translating a book on pharmacology that described Peruvian bark, a preparation made from a tree that was highly effective in treating malaria. As medicine in his era had no scientific basis, the only explanation offered by the textbook for Peruvian bark's curative effect was that it had the capacity to upset the stomach. It was a cockamamie time for the field of medicine. The most respected theory of the era was the doctrine of signatures, which a German mystic named Jacob

Boehme had popularized in two books, *Aurora* and *The Signature of All Things*, more than a century earlier.

The doctrine of signatures was a purely philosophic notion until Boehme's predecessor, the alchemist Paracelsus, had applied it to medicine. It postulated that certain features of a plant carry indications of its medicinal use. For example, plants with yellow roots or flowers (yellow signature) were supposed to cure jaundice. Plants impregnated with the color red (red signature) were considered to be beneficial for blood disorders. The hue of Iris resembled bruises, so that's what the plant was used to treat. Also the shape of plants played an important role in determining their uses.

Hahnemann couldn't accept the textbook's silly explanation for why Peruvian bark worked so well. He decided to take the preparation himself and find out what would happen. After a few repeated doses of Peruvian bark, he developed symptoms that closely resembled the symptoms of malaria. These subsided shortly after discontinuation of the medication. Hahnemann described this experiment in a footnote to the translation, which was published in 1790. Six years later, after a continuous literature search and further experimentation, Hahnemann published a landmark article, "Essay on a New Principle for Ascertaining the Curative Powers of Drugs." In this piece, he proclaimed the discovery of a curative law of nature: "*Similia similibus curentur*" ("Like cures like").

You were introduced to the principle of similars in the story about Tim's eczema. Let's look at another real present-day example to see how it operates. Yellow jasmine poisoning causes severe weakness with significant heaviness in the back of the head, heavy eyelids, and chills running up and down the back.[1] The homeopathic preparation of this flower, a remedy called *Gelsemium*, has shown to be very helpful for treating the flu in people who develop the same set of symptoms.

Superficially, it might seem as though the use of the conventional drug Ritalin for the treatment of attention-deficit hyperactivity disorder (ADHD) follows the principle of similars. Ritalin is a stimulant given to children who are restless to calm them. But the way the medication is typically used actually doesn't correlate with our natural law.

For a medication to be suitable for a specific patient, other individual characteristics must be present beside the ones that everyone exhibits. In the case of ADHD, as a common symptom is restlessness, we would look elsewhere. The same remedy won't work for everyone. Furthermore, remedies need to be homeopathically prepared—diluted and activated—a process described in detail in Chapter 3.

Another interesting modern example demonstrating the principle of similars is the conventional allergy elimination technique. First, an allergologist conducts a series of tests to find the allergen that's affecting someone. Then this same allergen is given to that individual in significantly smaller and smaller concentrations until the allergy goes away. Many children and adults have benefited from the application of this technique.

Interestingly, in the same year that Hahnemann published his seminal paper on homeopathy, British physician Edward Jenner published a paper on vaccination. He noticed that milkmaids never got sick with smallpox, a terrible, deadly infectious disease. But most of them had experienced cowpox, an illness benign to humans. Jenner cleverly suspected that milkmaids were protected from smallpox by having previously been exposed to the similar illness, thus he decided to inoculate people with cowpox to protect them from smallpox. In Latin, *vacca* means "cow." His idea worked perfectly. Thus, 1796 gave birth to two great medical discoveries, both of which incorporated the principle of similars.

Testing New Remedies

During his research on Peruvian bark, Hahnemann invented an experimental method for finding new remedies and investigating their qualities. He called this process a *prufüng*, meaning a "test." In English, it's known as a *proving*. Original provings were conducted using alcohol-based tinctures of various substances. Basically, he took the substance and then experienced a set of symptoms, which he recorded in great detail. Healthy volunteers, or *provers*, also received repeated doses of the substance in question, and then would describe all the symptoms they experienced.

Obviously, people have varying levels of sensitivity to particular substances and therefore develop different sets of symptoms depending on their individual dispositions. A few of the provers were highly sensitive to a particular substance and would develop hundreds, often thousands of symptoms. Other provers weren't sensitive to it at all.

A simple example of this very important idea is food sensitivity. You might know people who cannot drink coffee because they get headaches or feel jittery after taking even a sip or two of coffee. Such a person would be a perfect candidate for homeopathic proving of coffee as that person, who is so sensitive to coffee could develop many symptoms from even a minute dose of coffee. The same is true about people sensitive to certain odors.

I am sure, using this idea, you can easily continue making a list.

In reality, when a proving of a new substance happens, no one knows which person will wind up being sensitive to the substance under investigation. It is also remarkable to me that different people who are sensitive to the same substance will develop different reactions to it. In the example of coffee, one sensitive individual gets headaches, whereas another person feels jittery from imbibing coffee, but does not get a headache. This shows that the number of provers in a proving study has to be as big as possible because different provers will describe different aspects of having sensitivity to the same substance.

The systematic summary of everyone's combined symptoms is called *Materia Medica,* which is an old name for a textbook on pharmacology. It's a collection of descriptions of symptoms experienced by a pool of provers and also symptoms that arose during cases of accidental poisoning. At later points, symptoms which were discovered to be cured by the remedy that weren't in the original provings were also included in *Materia Medica.*

Provings were a prototype for the first phase in contemporary pharmacological studies of conventional drugs. There's a major difference between a proving and a phase one study, however. Phase one studies are designed to establish side effects. Homeopathic remedies don't have any "side" effects, however. All effects discovered in a proving are subsequently used to match a particular substance as closely as possible with the symptoms of a particular ill person. When a perfect match—in homeopathic parlance, the *simillimum*—is found, the remedy is administered to that sick person in order to stimulate a cure.

The questions I ask the people I am treating are intended to reveal their current simillimum. That's why my inquiry can go on for an hour and a half, like it did when I was speaking with Tim about his skin condition, or longer.

Double blind, placebo-controlled homeopathic provings already were routine by the early 1800s, whereas the first placebo-controlled study published by conventional medical researchers dates back to a 1948 trial conducted by the Medical Research Council on the use of streptomycin to treat pulmonary tuberculosis. The term *double blind* means that neither the participants nor the researchers in a study know which substance specific participants are receiving. The term *placebo-*

controlled indicates that an active substance—a medication of any kind—is being compared to a neutral substance, such as a sugar pill. Both requirements ensure that the results of an experiment are nonbiased.

Homeopaths instituted another important research design feature: the multicenter study. The importance of multicenter research is that it eliminates the influence of unforeseen variables, such as the character of a regional population and human error. If results are duplicated when conducting the same research in more than one location, it verifies that those results are extremely reliable and accurate. The first multicenter study of a homeopathic remedy (*Belladonna*) was conducted in 1906, whereas the first multicenter study of an allopathic drug was conducted in 1944.

I only present such facts to help you understand how the 200-year long feud between conventional physicians and homeopaths has translated into ignorance about homeopathy's scientific underpinnings. Unfortunately, our allopathic colleagues don't usually realize how deeply rooted homeopathy is in objective measures. Homeopathic prescribing is based on experimental data received from healthy humans. Its practice is rooted in precise and rational scientific observations.

During Hahnemann's research and professional practice, he continually refined his understanding of homeopathy and his methods. For a long time, Hahnemann used fairly concentrated tinctures of substances. For an unknown reason, he started to dilute remedies in proportions of 1:10 (called *decimal* and marked with the letter X) or 1:100 (called *centesimal* and marked with the letter C). Between each of a series of dilutions, he hit the tube against a thick book ten to twenty times. He called this process *potentization*.

Hahnemann believed that vigorous shaking helped to extract healing energy from the active substance in the remedy, a vital force that could produce a response in a patient's vital force. Frankly, we don't yet have a better explanation. But we do know that he discovered that higher serial dilutions provide deeper and longer lasting results than lower serial dilutions. He didn't "dream up" or theorize these results. He just followed the data he was objectively collecting from the numerous patients he treated. It wasn't unusual for him to administer remedies diluted 10^{400} times (known as a 200C dose) or more.

Today, the majority of contemporary homeopaths from North America, Great Britain, and India use ultramolecular dilutions, as Hahnemann did. But, interestingly, a large group of homeopaths from other countries successfully employ remedies that contain discernable concentrations of original source materials. These remedies are still prepared by dilution with potentization, but they are much less diluted. For example, you might see a remedy marked with the letter X. Thus, when they're taken, they require significantly more frequent repetition than higher dilutions. For instance, taking two to three doses a day for a duration of a month or more, as opposed to taking one dose every few months, or even years, for ultramolecular dilutions.

The concept of ultramolecular dilutions, although significant, is not central to homeopathy. It's more important to remember that during the process of serial dilution the tube is vigorously shaken, or *succussed*, between each step. Again, I must refer you to Chapter 3.

Extremely Safe and Gentle

Physicians are taught in medical school that it's better to do nothing than to take an action that might harm a patient. This is the guiding principle of medicine, and has been for 2,500 years. According to legend, Hippocrates, the renowned Ancient Greek physician known as the "father of medicine," was already telling his students "First do no harm." Unfortunately, we know too well from past experience that conventional medications almost always produce side effects—some mild and some severe. A cold remedy can make you drowsy. An antibiotic can upset your stomach, cause severe allergies, or destroy important friendly bacteria in your gut. We often accept minor side effects as the "price we must pay."

Homeopathic remedies are nontoxic because they are highly diluted substances. Furthermore, they have no "side" effects because the effects—all of them—are the reason a particular remedy matches a particular person. Occasionally, I'll receive a call from a frantic mother whose child has just ingested half a container of a 30C potency remedy. Each container holds about seventy pellets. Anyone familiar with basic math can understand that even if taken at once the entire contents couldn't possibly cause any complications. The active ingredient in a 30C remedy has been diluted 10^{60}. That's a ten with sixty zeros following it (10 x 10 x 10 . . . sixty times over). The additional ingredient in the pellet is sugar.

Homeopathy is safer than conventional medicine. Look, you receive instructions on correct usage when either an allopathic doctor or a homeopath prescribes medication to you. The crucial difference here is that if you correctly follow the instructions when you take a homeopathic remedy, nothing bad is going to happen. But even if you correctly follow a doctor's instructions when taking a conventional drug, it could have side effects.

The principle of safety has played a defining role in my own life. It was a cold Russian winter in 1984, and I was working as a family physician in Moscow. A doctor in our clinic called in sick, so I agreed to cover her home visits. It was a busy day for me, full of cases of common colds and bronchitis. As one of the addresses belonged to a close friend of mine, I left this visit for the end of my tour. It would be so nice to meet him and talk about the American science fiction and jazz music we both liked! Finally, I was at his home. I rang the bell. A beautiful young lady opened the door, the patient. She turned out to be my friend's sister, Natasha. I never knew he had such a beautiful sister!

After examining Natasha, I diagnosed her with a mild case of bronchitis and offered her a few choices. She could take herbal expectorants, conventional medication, or homeopathy. She'd heard homeopathy was very good, and was surprised that a local family physician knew about it. In Russia, homeopaths are highly respected and usually expensive. She was eager to try it. Because I liked her and she was my friend's sister, I volunteered to go and fetch the remedy for her. She was instructed to take one pellet three times a day. During our follow up appointment, Natasha admitted that the pellets were so little and tasted so delicious that eventually she took all those remaining at once.

The results were amazing. Whatever I gave her worked well. She was cured. We got married a few months later. Did Natasha's treatment have any side effects? Actually, it did. We eventually had two beautiful daughters together.

Hahnemann was firm on the principle of giving a single remedy to a patient at one time. Throughout his life, he fought against the practice of polypharmacy, or prescribing numerous medications to the same patient, a problem that persists in allopathic medicine. Adverse reactions to medications must often be attributed to drug interactions. Two hundred years of experience have shown that homeopathic clinicians who follow the principle of using a single remedy receive much better and longer lasting results.

Of course, finding the special remedy for a special person can sometimes be difficult. But the results are spectacular. Soon you'll see for yourself.

Consistently Proven Effective

The foremost benefit of homeopathy is its efficacy. In fact, the primary reason homeopaths are enthusiastic about what we do is that we are privileged to witness the miracle of a complete cure every day. Frankly, we never get used to it. Even after practicing homeopathy for more than twenty years, I'm still amazed at how quickly the human body can recover from a seemingly dangerous condition after the administration of a lone tiny pellet. At conferences and social gatherings, whenever several homeopaths are in the room, there's an endless exchange of stories about the numerous "little" cures they've seen for acute conditions, such as hives, colic, and poison ivy, and the "big," amazing cures they've seen for severe chronic illnesses, such as asthma and attention deficit hyperactivity disorder.

Its consistent success rate was the most important factor in making homeopathy popular in the early 1800s, and it has kept the practice of homeopathy alive in the United States since then despite conventional medicine's opposition to its principles and methods. Of course, every homeopathic practitioner has experienced failures, yet our outstanding success in curing both children and adults motivates us to continue our efforts to find the perfect remedy for those patients we couldn't help right away.

Samuel Hahnemann became a medical celebrity in 1799 due to an early success. Only three years after homeopathy's official discovery, an epidemic of scarlet fever swept Germany. Children were the main victims of the illness, which is a severe form of strep throat. Hahnemann achieved such impressive results in the treatment and prevention of this deadly illness that soon many allopathic physicians adopted his new approach and began praising homeopathy. The outcome was staggering. Ten physicians gave the homeopathic remedy *Belladonna* to 1,646 children for prophylaxis, or preventative treatment, and reported that only 123 developed the illness, whereas the morbidity rate in the untreated population surged as high as 90 percent! Subsequently, the Protomedicus of Prussia, a public health official comparable to the U.S. Surgeon General, declared the remedy effective and the government made the use of Belladonna for the prevention of scarlet fever mandatory. Today, the scope of this decision would be similar to having our government recommend homeopathy for the treatment of cancer or AIDS.

From its inception, homeopathy has been able to treat epidemics with impressive results, making the approach popular worldwide. In *The Logic of Figures,* first published in 1900, Thomas Bradford, M.D., a homeopath and historian, compared success rates from allopathic therapeutics with those from homeopathy. Here are some interesting statistics he put together.

- In 1813, following the defeat of Napoleon's army by the Russians, retreating French troops carried an epidemic of typhoid fever through Europe. When the epidemic hit Leipzig, Hahnemann saw 180 cases of typhus. He cured all but two, representing a 1 percent mortality rate. Conventional physicians reported a 30 percent mortality rate.
- In the European cholera epidemic of 1831–32, homeopathic hospitals had 7–10 percent mortality rates, while conventional physicians saw rates of 40 to 80 percent. As a result, a law forbidding the practice of homeopathy in Austria was dropped.

- In 1854, cholera broke out in London. The House of Commons asked for a report comparing various methods of treatment. Initially, homeopathic figures weren't included. According to the report, the mortality rate for patients under allopathic care was 59 percent. In response to an inquiry by the House of Lords, statistics for patients under homeopathic care were then provided. The mortality rate was only 9 percent.
- During the 1850s, several epidemics of yellow fever hit the southern United States. Today we know that mosquitoes transmit this disease. William Osler, a prominent physician of that era and author of the famous book *Systems of Medicine,* reported that the allopathic mortality rate from yellow fever was 15–85 percent. Homeopaths reported a mortality rate between 6 and 7 percent. In a similar epidemic in 1878, the mortality in New Orleans as reported by allopathic physicians was 50 percent. Homeopaths reported mortality of 6 percent for 1,945 cases.
- Children have always been easy targets for severe infectious diseases, and one of the deadliest of these was diphtheria. Although diphtheria was eventually eliminated by the advent of widespread vaccination, before then it was difficult to treat, as it rarely had the same presentation. Almost every case was a life or death proposition. Records from 1862 to 1864 in Broome County, N.Y., indicate an 84 percent mortality rate for patients given conventional medicine and only a 16 percent mortality rate for patients given homeopathy. Individualization of the homeopathic treatment was the most crucial factor in its success.
- Another devastating childhood disease is polio. Before the polio vaccine, this illness used to spread in epidemics, paralyzing and killing huge numbers of children. The most memorable outbreak was the infamous polio epidemic of the 1950s. An American

homeopath, Arthur Grimmer, M.D., and an Argentinean homeopath, Francisco Eizayaga, M.D., both reported excellent results from using homeopathy to prevent and treat polio prior to the introduction of the vaccine.

- In 1996, the Homeopathic Medicine Research Group, which was formed by the European Union to determine the effectiveness of homeopathy, conducted a large study. Importantly, scientists skeptical of homeopathy were involved in the design of the study. The study analyzed outcomes from seventeen clinical trials on a total of 2,001 subjects and showed that homeopathy was more effective than a placebo. There was only a slim probability (0.027 percent) that this result was due to chance.

The U.S. Centers for Disease Control and Prevention (CDC) estimates that 10–20 percent of Americans come down with the flu annually. Children are two to three times more likely than adults to get sick, and children frequently spread the virus to others. Although most people recover, the CDC estimates that more than 100,000 people in the United States are hospitalized and about 36,000 people die from the flu and its complications every year. Taking statistics into account, homeopathy is a significant untapped resource.

The flu pandemic of 1918–19 is still remembered for its devastating death toll. Considered one of the worst epidemics in U.S. history, with 600,000 people dead, it took the lives of 20–40 million people worldwide. In 1921, in a long article about the epidemic, *The Journal of the American Institute of Homeopathy* reported that in Dayton, Ohio, the overall mortality rate of flu patients was 28 percent, while in 26,000 cases of flu treated homeopathically patients had a mortality rate of only 1 percent. Hahnemann College in Philadelphia reported a similar figure for their homeopathic treatment of flu in 26,795 cases that year. Similar statistics came from other homeopathic physicians across the country. Flu season typically lasts from November to March. The media-generated panic that surrounds it each year keeps the memories of the earlier disaster alive.

Cases When Homeopathy Won't Work

Homeopathic treatment doesn't work in situations where structural damage has been done to a patient's body, cases such as genetic disorders, birth defects, and other profound physical conditions (such as side effects from conventional medication or certain types of injuries). In other words, a condition has an *obvious* cause that may or may not be reparable—but, if so, only by some means other than homeopathy.

Genetic Disorders and Birth Defects: Homeopathy cannot work if someone has a genetic disorder that's resulted in significant physical or emotional/mental deficiencies. For instance, children with Down syndrome have multiple health issues. Although many concerns can be relieved with homeopathy, defects related to intellectual functioning and structural changes of the cartilage cannot be removed. The same is true of other genetic disorders. They are inbuilt.

Pregnant women who consume significant amounts of alcohol or illicit drugs can damage their babies in the womb. These irreversible defects can be quite significant. Interestingly, when attempts are made to treat these children homeopathically, at first there's often a significant improvement in different levels of functioning. But eventually it trails off. The next prescription usually results in a less intense and shorter-lived response.

Side Effects of Medication: Frequently it's impossible to treat the side effects of a conventional drug with homeopathy. But there's a way around the problem.

Imagine that someone comes to the emergency room with a knife sticking out of his thigh and says, "Listen, Doc. You have to help me. But you cannot touch the knife!" Although it would be possible to give the guy painkillers, that type of care would be silly. To close the case, all you need to do is remove the knife and sew up the wound.

In the instance of treating side effects, my advice is to discuss possibly changing the medication with the doctor who prescribed it.

To be fair, I must admit that some homeopaths claim success in treating side effects of allopathic medications. At least one book has been published on this subject. Still, the proposition doesn't make as much sense as changing medications. Doctors have many drugs of the same type to choose from and can usually adjust their treatments.

Now, of course, an even more reasonable solution is to try to cure an illness with homeopathy rather than conventional means. If you succeed, then your child won't need allopathic medication. But is this true for every illness? What can homeopathy do for terrible chronic diseases, like cancer and AIDS, which don't spare children?

Advances have been made in the homeopathic approach to life-threatening, chronic illnesses. However, conventional physicians have been increasingly successful at saving and prolonging the lives of patients with cancer and AIDS. A significant amount of money has been directed toward the research and development of medications in these areas. Thousands of dedicated physicians and scientists have been working on saving people's lives. We cannot disregard these facts! As a parent, you should always consult with experts in the field before making a critical, life-altering decision.

Reversible Structural Problems: A few years ago, I received a referral patient from a famous homeopath. Noel, a slightly obese woman in her late fifties to early sixties, had been seen by this homeopath three times without success. She complained of excruciating pain in her right shoulder, and her story was quite remarkable. Noel claimed that while she was asleep, her husband, also a very large man, had rolled over in his sleep, pressed on her chest, and dislocated her right collarbone, thus causing all her subsequent pain.

Every conventional specialist possible saw her. Numerous imaging studies, including an MRI, had been performed. They found nothing. As happens very frequently when doctors don't find answers, Noel was pronounced "anxious," "depressed," or perhaps "psychotic." As a result, she was placed on many painkillers, mood stabilizers, and antidepressants. The list of her medications was long and scary. Certainly, she had many side effects from them, too. Although Noel *knew* that she was right, the doctors' studies just didn't support her claim.

Noel went to an acupuncturist. No results. Finally she located the famous homeopath. He prescribed a few remedies for her with no effect, and also decided that the woman was probably psychotic. That's when I came in handy, for I am a psychiatrist as well as a homeopath. In this case, I made the perfect "second opinion."

Noel came to see me along with her husband. The first thing I noticed was that they both were very honest, normal people, and Noel was suffering a lot. After taking a thorough history, I was convinced that there was no evidence of mental illness. I believed Noel's story. I also knew something that the conventional medical doctors refuse to admit to their patients, which is that there are *osteopathic* physicians. These doctors are specially trained to diagnose and treat structural changes, even if they are very minute.

I sent Noel to an excellent osteopath, who also saw nothing in the tests. But an osteopathic examination showed that her collarbone did move just a tiny bit. In an area so rich with nerve endings, this minute displacement was causing Noel an enormous amount of pain. The osteopath adjusted the problem. Literally, after the very first visit, Noel felt much better. For the first time in many years her pain was diminishing! In three to four weeks she was off most of her medication. She was cured!

This case illustrates a few important points. First, it proves—yet again—that our collective knowledge has many limitations, even when we use modern technology. Secondly, if there is an *apparent* cause of an illness, it has to be removed. Thirdly, do not give up on your convictions about your family's health. If you know why your child is ill, pursue the line of treatment that can remove the cause. Furthermore, medical miracles can happen. I know, for example, that osteopathic physicians adjust severely displaced collarbones in newborns. The results look like a miracle, but they're not. There are many other health care providers, both alternative and conventional, who can treat your child. Of course, I've seen many so-called miracles that happened with homeopathy.

A Holistic Approach

Homeopathy uses a holistic approach. Whereas an allopath looks at a patient in segments, as if under a microscope, and frequently forgets about the person as a whole organism, a homeopath looks at a patient through two lenses: a telescopic lens, to see the person's entire health picture, and a microscopic lens, to distinguish what makes this person unique. When we look at people as unified beings with a telescopic perspective, we begin to understand their true level of health.

Understanding levels of health is important. We need to know how healthy or sick we are so that we'll know what to expect from our treatment—homeopathic or otherwise—and what various symptoms indicate.

How frequently have you heard about someone with a serious illness who was told by doctors ten years earlier that he had less than a year to live? I'm guessing often. At least, I have. I used to laugh at scenes in movies and books in which a doctor somberly informs a patient, "You have three months to live." How would the doctor know? Who is this doctor, a god or something? I find prognoses of death unbelievable, especially when they come from allopathic physicians who are consumed by issues such as gross and cellular pathology, testing (of all kinds), and poisonous medications.

There is a way to see the big picture and it's actually rather easy to understand. That is, after a leading Greek homeopath of our era, George Vithoulkas, digested it all for us in his book *The Science of Homeopathy*.

Let's consider a human body as a system composed of overlapping concentric circles, resembling a dartboard. If we imagine these circles, which are growing in diameter, the innermost circle will represent the emotional/intellectual level, the second circle will represent the vital organs, and the outermost circle will represent the skin and other less important organs. According to this model, the inner circle is surrounded and protected by the outer circles.

This is also how it is in real life. Our mental and emotional functions are the most important ones. Without them, we don't exist. In order to provide sufficient housing and energy supplies to these functions, we need our vital organs—the brain, heart, lungs, stomach, liver, colon, and so forth. To create support and protect the vital organs, we need our skin, our skeleton, and all the other devices of our body. When a person is injured, the blood flow is naturally redirected to supply the vital organs first.

I think we can agree that the deepest dimension of our being is that of the emotional/mental self. Have you ever entered a room and instantly liked or disliked someone there without even talking to him? Think back to college or high school. Perhaps a new professor or student entered the classroom and—in a flash—you just knew you'd get along well. That's how quickly and deeply the emotional self works. When we're upset, we cannot function well in any capacity. Emotional pain can be as strong as physical pain or stronger. The mind is important, too. Without clarity of mind, everything else is irrelevant.

Next comes the dimension of the vital organs. We wouldn't be able to feel, think, or do anything if we didn't have a brain or a heart, or a set of lungs, a liver, and so on. Is this starting to remind you of *The Wizard of Oz?* Remember how important these dimensions were: The Cowardly Lion desperately needed courage (emotion), the Scarecrow needed a brain (vital organ), and the Tin Man wanted a heart (vital organ).

The least important, albeit still valuable, dimension of our being includes our skin, bones, and other more surface organs and attributes. Now, when the body aims to heal itself, it tries to express its problems at the most superficial level it can. This fundamental concept in homeopathy relates to the natural tendency of the human body to protect its vital core.

As a child, I went to school with boy named Michael who was intellectually delayed. He had a large head, but couldn't read, even in the fifth grade. While this lack of sufficient progress is sadly a reality for many students in America with normal intelligence, it was unheard of in Russia in the '60s and '70s unless a person was developmentally disabled. And Michael was. His behavior was offbeat, too. He often was putting his face close to someone else's, peering into the windows of apartments on the ground floor of buildings, and cursing. But, even during the frigid Russian winter, Michael walked around just in shorts and a tee shirt.

To the neighbors, his mother would sometimes say something along these lines: "Michael is not so smart, but at least he's healthy." *Wrong!*

Michael wasn't healthy. In fact, he was very ill. His most important functions were significantly impaired, although the housing for them (his brain) was pretty large. Please take your time to think about what I tell you next, as it is important. A smart, humorous teenager with terrible pimples is much healthier than a school beauty that sulks around and has suicidal tendencies.

Actor and director Christopher Reeve was one of the most astonishing examples of the accuracy of this three-level diagram of health. After the horseback riding accident that paralyzed him, he lost the use of his body, but retained his mind and his soul. At the core, he was healthier than thousands of good-looking, but totally dysfunctional junkies or severely developmentally disabled people, because his emotions and his intellect were intact! I'm not saying he didn't have bad days, as I'm sure he did. But he was resilient. He ultimately died because the structural damage to his body was too severe.

Of course, there are also cases when a physical illness adversely affects a person's emotional and mental state. This means that the person is deeply ill—malfunctioning on all three levels. I've met people with severe cases of cancer who were happy and I've met teenagers with pimples who were almost suicidal. The intimate interplay of various levels of our body and soul creates an opportunity to assess a person's future prospects. A child with severe pneumonia who's happy and surrounded by a loving family has a much better chance of a complete recovery than an unhappy orphan with eczema. In homeopathy, when we look at someone's symptoms, we take the mind/emotions/body into account.

This brings us to the discussion of a slightly different dimension of our health. Obviously, the severity of an illness significantly affects the whole person. Anyone who's had a toothache or a splitting headache will tell you that they felt totally miserable and absolutely couldn't function. I frequently hear statements along the following lines: "I'd rather have my hand amputated than have this terrible toothache" or "There's nothing worse than migraines!" People say such things in the heat of the moment. But how can we properly assess the level of health based on the severity of the illness?

We can actually distinguish four major levels of health.

Hering's Law: The Direction of Cure

First described in the works of Hahnemann, Constantine Hering, M.D., one of the founders of American homeopathy, clearly articulated a healing phenomenon that's now known as Hering's Law. This principle states that a homeopathic cure happens from the inside out, from the top of the body moving toward the bottom, and chronologically backward. It's as though you were watching a movie of your life in reverse, only faster, but only in terms of symptoms of disease. This natural principle was discovered during the observation of thousands of patients, and through the careful documentation of their chronological development of symptoms as well as of the way they went away after homeopathic treatment. Parents may notice it happening when their children improve the level of their health. It's a terrific sign of progress when it occurs.

Many years ago, I prescribed a homeopathic remedy for Boris, a twelve-year-old boy with ADHD and other severe behavioral problems.

Over the course of two months or so, Boris stopped hitting other children, he began paying more attention at school, and his teachers reported significant progress to his parents. However, even as Boris continued making strides academically and started having more friends, he also developed asthma. Boris' parents were extremely concerned. At our follow up appointment, they told me how disappointed they were with the "side effects" of the remedy.

We discussed the case. At first, they didn't grasp that the remedy Boris took more than two months earlier couldn't have been responsible for his asthma attacks since it was so highly diluted and was given only once. Then, I asked them if Boris had ever had the same symptoms before. The issue hadn't come up at his initial evaluation. Suddenly both parents said, "Aha!" They told me that when their son was four he had asthma, which was treated for a few years. Finally, after a course of prednisone, the asthma was gone.

I explained Hering's Law and reassured them that Boris' asthma would probably go away shortly. I also asked if there were any other illnesses they'd forgotten to mention. They recalled that at two Boris had many ear infections and sinus infections that required numerous courses of antibiotics before they "went away." They also told me that at twelve months he had severe diaper rash, especially in the front, and, later, some mild eczema that "went away" after a few applications of prednisone cream. Their report sounded like a common scenario for children from the late 1980s onwards.

These parents were intelligent and realized that all the former issues might return as a result of the homeopathic treatment Boris received. If so, I assured them that we'd be able to deal with each one successfully without too much pain. All the illnesses they'd mentioned seemed to fit nicely into the picture of the remedy I had given to Boris. Thus, in this case, all we needed to do was to repeat the remedy when it became necessary.

My prognosis was correct. The asthma was mild and went away rapidly. A few months later, Boris, who was still doing well emotionally, developed an ear infection. It was fairly significant, so I suggested he take a new dose of the same remedy. I know that infection went away, but I don't know what happened after the next year, as Boris was doing well and I lost track of him. Although his eczema didn't come back during the period in which I treated him, if it had I suspect it would follow a typical healing pattern. I've treated numerous cases of eczema and psoriasis. In general, but not always, the rash initially worsens somewhat. Afterwards, it clears first on the face, then on the torso and arms, and then it moves lower and lower in the body, until it disappears completely.

My eldest daughter's recovery from measles illustrates the direction of cure. First, her cough went away. Then, her rash cleared from her face, trunk, and arms. Finally, it cleared from her legs. The moment the rash cleared from her feet her fever came down.

In my days of conventional psychiatric practice, I often observed a similar direction of cure. But I'm not always able to persuade my patients that it's a sign of progress or to teach them how to take the opportunity to strengthen their immune system by forgoing interventions. One of my patients was suffering from severe, disabling depression. After completing a course of antidepressants, his depression went away. He then developed a severe bilateral ear infection. With my prompting, he remembered that something similar had happened many years earlier. He'd had a severe ear infection that was treated with antibiotics for a few months. To treat the reemergence of his ear infections, I suggested homeopathy. But he refused. Instead he chose to take a new course of antibiotics. His treatment took a long time. The ear infection subsided, but his mood became significantly worse. Despite my best efforts, it never improved to the extent it had before.

Sadly, we can see clearly that the direction of my psychiatric patient's treatment was wrong. According to the scheme we discussed above, the cure should have moved from the deepest level (his emotions/mind) to the periphery (in this case, his ears). Using conventional medications, such as antibiotics, suppresses symptoms and drives them underground, neutralizing this healing mechanism. Homeopathy supports the body to express symptoms and thus, essentially, to go back and complete necessary healing.

Unfortunately, there has been no funding available for a retrospective study of the thousands of children who received suppressive treatments for skin problems, like Boris' diaper rash and eczema, to see how "deep" the pathology goes. No one really knows why a particular child develops a skin disease. We say *predisposition* or *genetics*, but these are only words. Even if we were to identify a particular gene or group of genes responsible for asthma, we don't know what would happen if we altered them—maybe something better or maybe something significantly worse.

The bottom-line is that suppressive allopathic treatment of relatively superficial problems doesn't resolve a condition's underlying cause. The body has to deal with it the best it can, and it does by creating a new set of symptoms, usually on a deeper level. When a child or an adult shifts from one level of health to the next with the support of homeopathy, we are likely to see signs of former conditions that have been suppressed reemerging. In children whose immune responses haven't been suppressed with medications, such as my daughters, we see diseases expressed and healed according to the direction of cure. In this way, acute illnesses are not driven underground to take root as chronic illnesses.

Acute vs. Chronic Illness

Today, millions of people have chronic illnesses, such as ongoing series of ear infections and sinus infections. In November 2023, I conducted a basic internet search on the term *chronic disease*. Google turned up a few billion web pages. What's the reason chronic disease is so prevalent in our culture? Why are we facing an increase in disease? Simple. As I've already stated, conventional medicine provides suppressive treatment and transforms acute diseases into chronic ones. We are *all* chronically ill, and have been for a long time. But our children in particular are getting weaker. So let me begin to address this concern. Homeopathic theory understands this issue. As you'll see later in this book, homeopathy also can provide us with solutions.

Hahnemann was the first physician to classify diseases as acute or chronic. In his main work *Organon of the Medical Art,* he clearly defined them both. Let's examine his definitions and compare them to definitions embraced by conventional medicine.

Acute illness: Conventional physicians define acute illness as a condition that starts suddenly and is short lived. Homeopaths define it as a short-lived condition with symptoms that are *different* from the usual characteristics of the person, and different from the symptoms of any persistent condition the person has.

Acute illnesses have a few important characteristics. Specifically:
- Their onset is sudden.
- Their progress is rapid.
- They finish their course more or less quickly.
- They have a tendency to heal naturally (in other words, without intervention).

- Without treatment, they end in complete recovery or death. (Of course, these days death is an unlikely outcome for an acute illness.)

One of the most obvious examples of an authentic acute illness is an epidemic. Hahnemann actually distinguished individual, sporadic, and epidemic acute diseases. Individual disease doesn't require any explanation. Sporadic disease means a few people in different locations develop an acute illness with the same set of symptoms. During an epidemic, a large proportion of the population suffers from the same disease. If its causative agent is very strong, the majority of these people will have similar symptoms and may require the same homeopathic remedy. The existence of microscopic organisms such as bacteria, viruses, and fungal spores, was discovered during the period of 1665–83 by two fellows of the Royal Society of London, Robert Hooke and Antoni van Leeuwenhoek. In *Micrographia* (1665), Hooke presented the first published depiction of a microorganism, the microfungus Mucor.[2]

Symptoms of true acute conditions are usually prominent. If someone has an acute illness, you will be able to see the symptoms. Hopefully, if it happens to you or with one of your children you'll also give them what he or she needs to overcome the illness and remain healthy. In some cases, early symptoms of an illness can be seen only in the first couple of hours. This phenomenon provides parents a great opportunity to halt the disease in its tracks. I know of many cases when this has happened. This book will teach you how to perform this miracle, using homeopathy, for the great benefit of your family, friends and children.

Chronic illness: Conventional physicians define a chronic illness as any disease that develops slowly and lasts a long time. Homeopaths also define it as a long-lasting condition; but they emphasize that when it flares up it may resemble an acute illness. Its symptoms will be the same every time there's an episode, just pronounced.

Importantly, according to homeopathic theory a chronic illness is not self-limiting. If left untreated or treated allopathically, sooner or later it will get worse.

Before we delve any deeper into these two categories of illness, let's see how important the distinctions between them can be in real life. Imagine that Dr. Watson was magically transported to our day and age. He saw many patients today. Two boys, Sherlock Holmes and Alexander Moriarty, left the most remarkable impression. Both had come down with ear infections a week ago and were seen by the doctor immediately. He gave penicillin to each. Today, their parents brought them in for follow up visits. Young Sherlock was cured. He had no pain and showed no signs of inflammation during his ear exam. Clearly he is a happy healthy lad.

By way of contrast, Alexander's parents reported that although he had no fever, their son was weak and complained of discomfort in his ear. On examination, there were still signs of inflammation. Dr. Watson had to give Alexander another prescription for a different antibiotic. The poor Moriartys! Their unfortunate son has been having those stubborn ear infections for a few years already.

As you have probably guessed, although their symptoms were similar, Sherlock had an acute ear infection, whereas Alexander actually had an *exacerbation* (a medical term for the worsening) of a chronic illness. Sherlock is at Level 1 of health, as he doesn't have any chronic problems. Alexander is at Level 2 of health, as he has a recurring problem. According to what homeopaths believe, homeopathic treatment would have been better for the boys than penicillin, because it strengthens all the defense mechanisms of the body. Even with the medication, and perhaps because of similar courses of medication in the past, Alexander has developed chronic otitis media. So he's probably going to have an ear infection, presenting with a similar combination of symptoms, every time he's subjected to a significant stressor like cold weather, emotional trauma, or a virus.

What could his parents do to help young Alexander regain his health? They need to help him fight his illness all the way through to the end so he can get rid of his current predisposition to ear infections. This requires professional homeopathic help. Imagine what could have happened if Alexander was treated homeopathically the first time he had an acute cold or flu that turned into otitis media. It would be over!

The problem with conventional treatment is that it suppresses the body's symptoms. Although it seems like the illness goes away, in reality the root of the problem is not being addressed. Only individuals who are at Level 1 of health are cured. But even for them, the unnecessary use of antibiotics is detrimental. Antibiotics always weaken the immune system and in time move a child from Level 1 health to Level 2 health.

Don't get me wrong. I strongly believe that antibiotics must be used when necessary. Fortunately, in the majority of cases, natural treatment modalities, such as homeopathy, are good enough and antibiotics are unnecessary. Homeopathy helps to make us stronger and more independent. Homeopathic physicians believe that allopathic drugs make patients depend on them more and more by virtue of transforming acute problems into chronic ones. That being said, we need to be very much aware of the main principle of medicine: FIRST CAUSE NO HARM. Safety always has to come first.

I urge you strongly to remember that there is a window of opportunity for homeopathy to come in before something else needs to be done. For example, if you were involved in an accident that in your opinion requires homeopathic *Arnica* (described in Chapter 9) and you have it with you, take it on your way to the emergency room or urgent care or your doctor. If your child developed an ear infection and the doctor decided to practice watchful waiting for a day or two, that is how much time you have to try a homeopathic or any other natural way of healing. If it worked, and the doctor gave your child a clean bill of health—then great. If not, you should be prepared to give antibiotics. Not doing so may result of severe medical problems including generalized infections and/or loss of hearing.

There is no reason to take a stand against antibiotics as long as they are used rationally when indicated. If this is the only message you get from this book, I will be perfectly happy. My goal here is to provide you with a description of possible natural solutions you could use WHILE YOU ARE ON THE WAY TO RECEIVE PROFESSIONAL HELP.

The majority of people who live in industrial societies nowadays are at Level 2 of health. They are much more vulnerable to developing chronic problems than earlier generations were. Back in his era, Hahnemann noticed some cases in which even the best outcomes of treatment didn't last a long time. He suggested that certain people—now the majority of our population—are predisposed to chronic illnesses since birth. He called this predisposition a *miasm*. Perhaps it's a viable explanation for what's happening to contemporary children and adults.

The Theory of Miasm

Hippocrates (circa 460–370 BCE) was the first physician to use the term *miasm* to describe an infectious agent. The concept has its origins in the Greek word for "taint" or "fault." He postulated that diseases could be transmitted to humans through tainted air and water. After rediscovering the writings of Hippocrates, eighteenth-century physicians adopted the belief that impure airs were responsible for the spread of epidemic diseases. Although Samuel Hahnemann agreed that air could carry infectious diseases, he didn't consider the pathogenic material to be gaseous in nature. For instance, he realized that syphilis was a contagious blood disease that could mask itself behind the symptoms of many different illnesses.

Hahnemann redefined Hippocrates' miasmatic approach. After twelve years of thorough clinical observation and historical research, he published a new theory in his book *The Chronic Diseases* in 1828.

According to Hahnemann, all diseases result from inherited predispositions. He insisted that specific morbid tendencies are passed from one generation to the next, and he used the term *miasmatic animalcule* in reference to how they were transmitted. *Animalcule* means an "animal invisible to the naked eye." Dutch naturalist Antonie van Leeuwenhoek invented the microscope and had published his observations of small living animalcules (microbes) before his death in 1723. Hahnemann, although obviously thinking about microorganisms in regard to miasms, didn't know about DNA or genetics. In his book, he offered numerous examples that unequivocally supported his theory.

Originally, Hahnemann identified three major types of miasms. He gave them metaphoric names: the *psoric* (derived from the Greek word *psora*, meaning "itch"), the *sycotic* (derived from the Greek word *syco*, meaning "fig"), and the *syphilitic*. By *syphilitic* (derived from a Greek myth about a shepherd punished by the gods), Hahnemann did not mean the sexually transmitted disease.[3] Although each type of miasm clearly applies to particular diseases, the true essence of the theory of miasm is that people are prone to developing particular sets of problems. Miasms are responsible for diseases of a chronic nature, and also lay a foundation for all disease in general. An individual can have any number from one to all three of these major predispositions.

Some of the basic characteristics of these three miasms are:

Psoric. The entire population shares this predisposition, as it is the most ancient and established a foundation for all other miasms. Its main characteristics are a constant feeling of lack, a need to get more, and a need to be surrounded with more and more protection. This tendency materializes on every level of the human being: anxiety, fears, feeling cold (lack of heat), weakness (lack of strength), conservation, and a constant "itch." Those who were born with a prevalence of psoric features often are plump; cry a lot; have many fears; like to be pampered; like "comfort foods," such as milk, eggs, and pastry; need additional layers of clothes; and prone to frequent skin itchy eruptions.

Sycotic. This miasm represents excess, the need to connect, and the need to spend—a tendency that manifests itself in all the dimensions of the human being, too. People who possess this miasm tend to be extremely sociable and sexual; love animals; have more energy at night; have physical problems that manifest with excess, such as discharges, skin growths; and feel warm most of the time. As their name suggests, sycotic eruptions resemble little figs. Warts are a good example of these.

Syphilitic. The main characteristic of this miasm is destruction—aimed outwardly and inwardly. To repeat: It is not a reference to a sexually transmitted disease. I hope none of the people you know or your children is born with pronounced syphilitic tendencies. These children are prone to behaviors such as torturing animals, and teasing or tormenting their siblings. They may also be self-destructive, possibly depressed and even suicidal—sometimes at a very young age. Syphilitic physical problems would include bleeding ulcers and such.

Let me reiterate, microbes do *not* cause the miasms. The theory of miasm could be considered another, more exotic way of talking about genetics that was introduced before actual discovery of genetics and DNA. According to homeopathic theory many generations ago, microbes and possibly other influences—we don't know exactly what—caused changes in our ancestors. These morbid, or unhealthy, tendencies (miasms) were then passed along to their descendants from one generation to the next. Thus a familial predisposition was created to react to significant stressors *of any kind* in a predictable way.

If an individual with pronounced sycotic tendencies were exposed to gonorrhea, symptoms would flourish quickly in that person. But only a small percentage of people exposed to gonorrhea go on to acquire the miasm. They're either born with it or not. It would take substantial exposure to acquire a new miasm of any kind. Of course, once it did set in, a miasm would be passed on to all succeeding generations.

A common misunderstanding about this theory is to believe that the different miasms are assigned to particular illnesses. In reality, *any* illness can represent various miasmatic tendencies. It just depends on what stage is the illness in. For example, a person suffering from depression may be uncommonly anxious at the onset of the illness, reflecting a psoric stage. Then the person may become extremely irritable, reflecting a sycotic stage. Finally, if the depression is left untreated, this individual might develop strong suicidal tendencies, which would represent a syphilitic pathology.

Our understanding of miasms has expanded since Hahnemann's day. Presently, homeopaths distinguish as many as ten different miasms. What's important for you to understand, 'is that the theory of miasma is groundwork for how homeopathy is practiced. It is a partial explanation for why numerous layers of illness may be present in the same individual.

Any time chronically ill patients come to me for treatment, I know that their multiple layers of disease probably were created not as much by their miasmatic predispositions as by other modern problems, such as:

- Attempts to suppress symptoms of past acute illnesses with allopathic drugs.
- Side effects of medications.
- Unreasonably aggressive vaccination schedules.
- The high level of daily stresses provided by the modern lifestyle.

The majority of homeopathic practice is devoted to "peeling off" multiple layers of illness if they exist. The ultimate goal is always to restore Level 1 health. In the next chapter, we'll explore how homeopathic remedies are made, and you'll begin to understand how the principles we've been discussing can very effectively, and easily, be put to use.

Constitutional Treatment

Identifying the correct remedy for a chronic condition is a different and more complicated process then finding a remedy for an acute ailment. To find any remedy, homeopaths need to know what changes—characteristic to this particular person—have been caused by a particular illness. In acute conditions, changes usually are obvious because they are new and strong. The integrative systems of our bodies try to externalize problems to protect the most important vital organs and systems. Symptoms are easy to recognize, and a relatively limited number of remedies tend to be useful.

Cocculus and Tabacum are most frequently indicated for the treatment of car sickness. The majority of people will exhibit signs and symptoms of these remedies, and only a smaller population will require alternatives. Similarly, the majority of the population will respond very well to either Apis or Ledum when stung by an insect, and only a smaller group will exhibit signs and symptoms of a few other remedies.

We can also look at the situation from the deeper perspective of homeopathic philosophy and say that a person who has responded to stress with certain signs and symptoms in one event, most probably will have a similar systemic response to any severe stressor. These stressors could be of an emotional nature (for example, a natural disaster, a terrorist attack) or a physical nature (for example, a severe infection, a severe trauma, surgery, having a baby). A stress is still a stress. The symptoms might be panicky: severe fear with a feeling of imminent death, accompanied by restlessness, heat, an expression of extreme fear on the face, and an unquenchable thirst for cold drinks.

A relatively healthy individual has a limited repertoire of symptoms that develop in response to various types and degrees of acute stressors. So a particular "melody" from this repertoire is played depending on what demand is being placed on the person at a particular time. Different people have different repertoires. That's why two people exposed to the same stressful event-for example, an earthquake-react in two ways. Let's say one goes into an *Aconitum* state (characterized by extreme agitation and panic), another into a *Gelsemium* state (characterized by extreme weakness and paralyzing anxiety).

If left untreated, these two individuals may either recover on their own without any trace of problems, or they may go into a deeper pathological state with more and more symptoms created on the emotional and physical levels. Diseased states have a tendency only to get worse, with pathology going deeper and deeper. The reality of our era is that by the time a sick person meets a homeopath, a number of other health professionals were already involved in that individual's treatment. A number of opportunities to address the problem when it was still relatively superficial were missed. The past use of suppressive methods of treatment makes the deciphering of the code of the illness even more difficult. It also alters and complicates the mechanisms used by the person's body for its healing response. Layers and layers of issues with their own patterns of response to various stressors have been superimposed on whatever remaining original, healthy, self-regulating mechanisms there are.

Because the person is now chronically ill, the changes the homeopath must identify can be extremely subtle, and the process of choosing the right remedy is laborious. Even in cases when a very well-known remedy is indicated, symptoms may not be as clear and straightforward as we might hope. The process of finding the correct remedy in these situations requires a deep understanding of the main principles of homeopathy, combined with clinical experience and detailed knowledge of homeopathic pharmacology. In this type of prescribing-that is, constitutional treatment-the homeopath attempts to find the remedy that will initiate a healing process on the deepest, constitutional level of the entire person.

Frequently, the path to the ultimate remedy requires consecutive prescriptions of other remedies. Each one peels off another layer of problems. It addresses problems that are the most current and disturbing to the mind-body continuum of the patient and therefore the most apparent to the homeopath. Afterward, another layer of problems emerges that requires a different remedy. Each remedy the homeopath selects should be precise and aimed at opening a passageway to the next level of illness and healing.

Even the most experienced homeopaths can face significant difficulties navigating the obstacles of the healing process. As a parent, you shouldn't attempt this type of treatment on your own. Just to give you a brief example, a few years ago, I saw a sixteen-year-old girl named Becky. She told me that she'd run away from home and gone to another state, where she was supposed to meet with representatives of the Mafia, because the CIA, FBI, and a few other important U.S. government agencies wanted her to penetrate it and provide them with information. The mission was so important that Becky lost sleep. But although she was hardly sleeping at all, she still had a lot of energy.

As you can tell, Becky was delusional. The episode had been triggered by the news that her grandmother was becoming progressively ill. Becky loved her grandmother very much. Grandma lived in the city where Becky went to "penetrate the Mafia." "When they found her missing, Becky's family had called the police, who were able to catch up with Becky quickly. She was hospitalized in the local psychiatric ward, stabilized on three medications, and then allowed to come home. That's when I met her.

Becky didn't want to take medication for several reasons. First, she was just being a teenager. And she felt good in her delusional state. Second, while on the drugs, her periods were irregular, which was upsetting. Third, Becky read that the medications would cause significant weight gain. That did it. She told her parents that she would have to stop taking them. The parents heard of me and brought Becky to my office.

One of the amazing symptoms that I noticed during the interview was that Becky suffered from psoriasis, a chronic skin disease that's characterized by a particular type of itchy rash. Large areas of her body were covered with the rash. But Becky told me that ever since she'd been "hired by the CIA," the itching had stopped. To me, her situation was obvious. The focus of Becky's problems was much deeper than her skin. It was in the core of her being-at the emotional and mental level. Becky had bipolar disorder.

After a few months of constitutional homeopathic treatment, Becky was able to discontinue taking two out of three of her conventional medications. She remained well. Even though she was a teenager and going to college, Becky did her best over the next several years to follow my directions concerning her lifestyle. Since then, she graduated college and got married. Now we're working together on getting her off her last allopathic medication. She hasn't had any symptoms of mania or depression in all of these years, even under the stress of planning a wedding!

As Becky was getting better, her psoriasis began to itch again. There were also other, new symptoms that led me to prescribe a different remedy. The psoriasis improved by about 80 percent. We hope that after discontinuation of the last conventional drug, Becky's body will be able to get rid of psoriasis completely.

In a way, the difference between the homeopathic treatment of acute and chronic illness is similar to learning a new language. Most of us can navigate ordinary situations during a brief vacation in a foreign country after learning a limited number of words and phrases in a strange language. We don't really need a deep understanding of grammar. We can get by after learning a few basic things about the culture and customs. If we don't understand an answer, we only have to turn to a tour guide for help. Homeopathy for most acute conditions isn't hard to handle, as you'll soon learn in Part Two. If you can't figure it out or you make a mistake, you can always zip over to the ER or phone a doctor.

Constitutional treatment is more like living in a country on a long-term basis. It's a totally different ball game. For that, we need to know the language and culture well. We need to be prepared to react appropriately to every possible situation that we might face. If we didn't have those abilities, we'd have to turn to a knowledgeable guide or partner. In constitutional treatment, homeopaths are the guides and the partners.

CHAPTER THREE

How Homeopathic Remedies Are Made and Regulated

"Good things come in small packages."
—AESOP

Remedies are the most important tools of homeopathy secondary only to homeopath's diagnostic and clinical skills. They are the catalysts of healing. Without them, there would be no homeopathy, for, as you already know, the basic principle of our approach is "like cures like." To produce a powerful effect, however, remedies must be prepared and taken according to a strict set of standards. In this chapter, you'll primarily learn how homeopathic remedies are made, but I will also explain how to use them in a safe and efficient way, and describe a special technique for dosing young children who can't take remedies in pellet form.

Before we move on to the specific instructions, let's address a foundational issue: regulation.

How Remedies Are Regulated

Homeopathic remedies have always been at the center of the controversy that surrounds homeopathy. Most M.D.s, and a significant fraction of the general public, have ridiculed the method of using highly diluted substances to promote healing since remedies were introduced. Michael Quinn, a well-known and respected American homeopathic pharmacist, writes: "[*the methods of homeopathic pharmacy*] have been both a blessing and a curse upon homeopathy to this day. [*They*] are a blessing because they allow us to prepare medicines of great efficacy and low toxicity; they are a curse because a practice of drastically diluting medicines appears so irrational..."[1]

Surprisingly, many people think that practitioners make homeopathic remedies themselves. They don't realize that homeopathic pharmaceutical companies in the United States and overseas are monitored for quality and adherence to specific, government-mandated procedures. In the United States, homeopathy is regulated by the Food and Drug Administration (FDA), which recognizes homeopathy as a legal product.

"Quack busters" frequently accuse homeopaths of sneaking homeopathy into national legislation. Here's the truth. Senator Royal Copeland of New York was chief sponsor of the 1938 Food, Drug, and Cosmetic (FDC) Act that paved the way for the establishment of the modern FDA. To this day, critics of homeopathy still refer to Copeland as the "prominent homeopathic physician," because he was a homeopathic medical doctor and served as president of the AIH in 1908. More interested in administration than in practice, he worked as a dean of New York Homeopathic Medical College from 1908 to 1923, and also as Health Commissioner for the City of New York from 1918 to 1923. In 1923, he was elected to the U.S. Senate, where he served until his death.

When Copeland introduced the first bill for a complete revision of the obsolete 1906 Food and Drugs Act into the Senate some ninety years ago, it launched a five-year legislative battle. The battle turned its course in 1937 after an antibacterial drug called elixir of sulfanilamide, containing a poisonous solvent, killed 107 people, most of whom were children. This event dramatized the need to establish stronger drug safety laws, which until then had been successfully and continuously resisted by the drug industry.

The 1938 FDC Act included the following provisions:

- Requiring new drugs to be proven safe before marketing, thus instituting a new system of drug regulation.
- Authorizing standards of identity, quality, and fill-of-container for foods.
- Authorizing factory inspections.
- Eliminating a requirement to prove intent to defraud in drug misbranding cases.
- Providing that safe tolerance levels would be set for unavoidable poisonous substances.
- Adding the legal recourse of court injunctions against violators to the previous penalties of seizures and prosecutions.
- Extending regulations to cover cosmetics and therapeutic devices.

The FDC Act also recognized the *United States Pharmacopeia* (USP) and the *Homeopathic Pharmacopeia of the United States* (HPUS) as official compendiums. The spirit behind it was to create strict standards for regulating drugs, food, and cosmetics. Both volumes contain definite instructions of how to manufacture medicinal products. We'll explore the homeopathic procedures designated by HPUS in a few pages.

Senator Copeland did not "sneak" anything into legislation. His homeopathic background helped him to clearly understand the need for strict standards for both homeopathic and allopathic medications, and prompted him to take a leadership role in advancing the cause of public safety. As you can see, these very important provisions created a solid foundation for what we know as the modern FDA.

What's on the Label of a Remedy?

Let's take a look at the label of *Arnica montana,* one of the most commonly used homeopathic medications. It reads:

> *ARNICA MONTANA 30CH*
> **HPUS**
>
> **HOMEOPATHIC MEDICINE**
> **ACTIVE INGREDIENT:** listed above.
>
> **USE:** for self-limiting conditions listed below • or as directed by a doctor.
>
> **WARNING:** Do not use if pellet-dispenser is broken. • **Stop use and talk to a doctor** if symptoms persist for more than 3 days or worsen. • **If pregnant or breast-feeding,** ask a health care professional before use. • **Keep out of reach of children.**

> **DIRECTIONS** (adults/children): At onset of symptoms dissolve 5 pellets in the mouth 3 times a day • or as directed by a doctor.
>
> **TRAUMA. BRUISES. MUSCLE SORNESS.**
>
> **Expiration date:** May 2028

New guidelines for homeopathic remedies were established in 1988 and enacted in 1990. According to these rules, homeopathic remedies are divided into two categories: over-the-counter (OTC) and prescription-only. The next point is *very important.* To be classified as OTC, a remedy must be labeled with an indication for the so-called self-limiting conditions it treats. There's a list of forty-five self-limiting categories. For example, on the *Arnica* label, we read: "Trauma, Bruises, and Muscle Soreness."

The situation resulting from the OTC guidelines can create a lot of confusion in patients' minds. Why? A given homeopathic remedy may have up to a few thousand indications. It's impossible to list them all on the product label. Also, most of the conditions a remedy cures, problems like depression or asthma, aren't self-limiting. They persist for a lifetime. Frequently, a patient buys the remedy from the health-food store and is deeply concerned that the indications on the container have nothing to do with the main complaint they had.

Here's an example from my private practice. In the beginning of my career as a homeopath in the United States, I saw an elderly lady with a number of mild neurological problems. The selection of the remedy was not difficult. I clearly saw that I had to prescribe *Causticum,* a remedy first introduced by Hahnemann that's made from a mineral. Among other serious systemic conditions, it's used to treat various neurological conditions. I prescribed the remedy and the lady went to get it. After she read the indication on the label, the lady became very upset and called me to say how disgusting I was for mocking her. The indication on the label was bedwetting! Bedwetting is one of a few thousand symptoms that can be helped with *Causticum,* as well as by many other, much more frequently indicated remedies.

Ever since this awkward incident, I explain to each of my new patients what I just told you. Still I'll frequently get a phone call from a concerned mother, who tells me, "I brought my son for treatment of his migraine and poor attention, and you prescribed a remedy for nasal discharge." And then I explain again: Homeopathic remedies are prescribed for the illness in the *particular individual,* not just for a diagnosis.

Please remember this point when you go to purchase a remedy suggested by your homeopath, and also when you shop for remedies on our own. Hundreds of remedies are potentially indicated for particular conditions depending on the individual characteristics of the intended recipient—you, your family member, or another patient. Homeopathy treats people, rather than diseases. Nonetheless, regulations require labels to list some conditions.

In accordance with FDA regulations, the label for an OTC remedy has to contain four more pieces of information.

- The concentration of the medication
- Instructions for its use
- Safety warnings
- The expiration date

So far we already understand a few things. We know the name of the remedy, which is written in Latin. All remedies have Latin names. This makes communication between homeopaths from different countries easy and maintains a clear standard for the sources of the remedies. But what does 30CH after the name of the remedy mean? We know that the acronym *HPUS* indicates that the remedy was manufactured according to the standards of the *Homeopathic Pharmacopeia of the United States.* We also know the use. What about the directions, the warning, and the expiration date?

The Making of a Remedy

In order for homeopathy to be effective medicine, remedies must be highly reliable. The preparation of homeopathic remedies—the way they are manufactured—is done in the same way around the world. The homeopathic pharmacopeias of various countries vary extremely little from each other, as there's a worldwide standard for each remedy. This includes the description of the raw material that goes into a remedy, the method and time of collection of this material, and the manufacturing process that's responsible for the accurate and consistent preparation of the remedy.

Homeopathic remedies have been prepared in the same manner ever since 1799, the year Hahnemann finalized the process for making them. Currently, 2,500–3,000 homeopathic remedies are produced from five major sources: minerals, plants, animals, disease tissue (aka *nosodes),* and conventional drugs. According to the standards and regulations established by the FDA, a new remedy must be demonstrated efficacious in homeopathic practice before it is accepted for inclusion in the HPUS. In other countries, homeopathic remedies are regulated only according to their preparation. Efficacy is frequently disregarded.

If interested, you can watch a demonstration of how homeopathic remedies are prepared on my YouTube Channel, @WiseMedicine.

The process of the preparation of a remedy consists of a few standard steps, as follows.

Step 1: The preparation of the so-called *mother tincture* (denoted by the Greek letter θ). This is a relatively concentrated, alcohol-based solution of the substance.

Step 2: Dilution of the mother tincture in a water-alcohol (ethanol) mixture.

Step 3: Potentization, or activation, of the remedy by *succussion*. Derived from a combination of the German word *schütteln* and the Italian word *scossone*, both meaning to "jolt" or "shake violently," succussion is a process during which the vial containing the solution is vigorously shaken. Substances that are diluted without being succussed do not share the same healing property as potentized substances.

Steps 2 and 3 are repeated to achieve a higher *attenuation* (dilution) and greater therapeutic strength. The final product of the process of attenuation is therefore identified as a specific *potency*. For example, you might say: "I am looking for *Arnica montana* in potency 30C (or 6X)." In homeopathy, potency is different than concentration. A preparation containing a higher concentration of source material would actually be of a lower potency than one that's more diluted.

The number with a letter listed on the label informs us about how many steps of attenuation and how many succussions were performed to achieve a particular potency.

The most frequently used homeopathic potencies are *decimal* (from the Latin word for "ten") and *centesimal* (from the Latin word for "one hundred"). In Latin, numerals are expressed with letters. Ten is represented with an X. One hundred is represented with a C.

In some European countries you may also find decimal dilutions marked with a D.

In the case of centesimal dilutions, such as in our *Arnica montana*, the dilution at each step is 1:100. Therefore, by the time the attenuation of 30C is reached, the remedy has been succussed 300 times and is diluted 10^{60} times.[2]

According to Avogadro's number—which is a formula used by chemists to calculate the number of molecules in a given amount of any chemical substance—the original substance in a homeopathic remedy disappears at the potency 12C (dilution 10^{24}).[3]

In the case of decimal dilutions, the dilution at each step is 1:10. 12X, for example, means that the remedy was diluted twelve times, succussed 120 times, and the degree of dilution is 10^{12}.

The *Arnica montana* label in the United States reads "30CH." What does the letter H stand for? It means "Hahnemannian." There are two main methods of homeopathic attenuation: Hahnemannian and Korsakovian. Samuel Hahnemann changed the vial at each step of his attenuation process. By contrast, General Semjon Korsakoff, a Russian homeopath, suggested using the same vial for all the steps. In Korsakovian attenuation, every subsequent dilution is achieved by emptying the vial of 99 percent of the previous attenuation, refilling it with fresh solvent, and then repeating the succussion process.

"CH" indicates centesimal attenuation, Hahnemannian style.

"CK" indicates centesimal attenuation, Korsakovian style. Semyon Korsakov was a famous homeopath who worked in the early nineteen century.

Usually Hahnemannian attenuation is used for the first 12–200 steps in preparing a remedy. Korsakovian method is typically used for higher attenuations.

Preparing Remedies from Insoluble Matter

Hahnemann developed a process that allows us to convert insoluble materials, such as metals like gold or platinum, into a form that can be introduced into the core process described above. This process is called *trituration*.

During this process, the insoluble substance is "diluted" with nine (or ninety-nine) times its weight of lactose (milk sugar). Trituration used to be performed by processing the mixture by hand using a mortar and pestle. Each step had to be performed for at least an hour. Modern homeopathic facilities now utilize a ball mill instead. This device consists of a cylindrical porcelain jar with a tight lid. The materials are placed in the jar together with very hard porcelain cylinders. The closed jar is then placed on horizontal rollers and rotated by electric motors for approximately two hours at each step.

After two triturations, the resulting remedy, now concentration 3C, goes into the core process. Now, operations are part of the usual cycle of homeopathic attenuations.

Extremely High Attenuations

The majority of homeopaths use remedies in centesimal and decimal potencies. Although decimal dilutions do not go higher than 200X, centesimal dilutions can go significantly higher. There are special ways to mark these very high attenuations. The dose 1000C is marked as 1M. Consequently, 10M = 10,000C. 50M = 50,000C. 100,000C = CM, and 1,000,000C = MM.

There's another variation that's marked as LM. Technically, LM1 = 1:50,000. During the preparation of LM potencies 1:500 dilution step is added to 1:100 step of the centesimal process. This way the ratio achieved at each step of the LM dilution is 1:50,000. These dilutions are succussed one hundred times at each step. LM potencies have been becoming more popular in the last ten to fifteen years. The proponents of LM potencies report significantly gentler actions of the remedies.

Making the choice of a particular potency is based on numerous and often complicated factors that should be left up to the professional homeopath. In your own small "family practice," you'll be safe using 30C and, in some cases, 200C potencies. We'll talk about those in Part Two of this book.

Pellets, Liquids, Ointments, and Gels

Homeopathic remedies are usually prepared in either pellet or liquid form (tinctures). The pellets are more popular, and generally easier to store and dispense. Their base material is a mixture of sucrose and lactose. They are safe for chemically sensitive individuals and diabetics. Best of all, children love these sweet little pills! The tinctures have an alcohol base, and therefore taste slightly bitter.

Pellets are medicated according to a strict protocol. For example, to prepare a pellet form of *Arnica montana* 30C, an 88 percent alcohol solution of the remedy is added to the pellets in a 1 percent ratio. We use 88 percent solutions, because if the concentration of alcohol were to be less than that, the water in the solution would dissolve the sugar pellets. In our case, 10 milliliters of the solution of *Arnica montana* 30C is added to 1,000 grams of sugar pellets. The pellets are thoroughly shaken to distribute the solution evenly. The pellets are soaked for five minutes, and then dried and packaged. Now the pellets contain *Arnica montana*

30C. Containers with pellets usually hold about 80 pellets of the standard size.

In addition to pellets and tinctures, homeopathic remedies are also produced in the forms of ointments, lotions, and gels, which can be applied externally. These have less therapeutic effect than internally consumed remedies. Furthermore, consumers can buy homeopathic suppositories and tablets. We'll discuss the administration of these forms of remedies as the book unfolds.

Expiration Dates

Although putting an expiration date on the container is required by FDA regulations, experience shows that homeopathic pellets and tinctures remain active for generations. Remedies made in the time of Hahnemann still exist and are effective. We know activity of more contemporary products is retained for several decades.

A Little Poison May Cure

The vast majority of parents are unconcerned about the source of homeopathic preparations. They're OK with whatever remedy the doctor chooses. Others become anxious and uncomfortable when they hear names like *Arsenicum, Carcinosin, Tarentula,* or *Tuberculinum.* The traditional folk names of some of the ingredients in homeopathic remedies don't necessarily sound nice and safe either. Wolf's Bane (*Aconitum*), for example, used to be used as a poison on the tips of hunters' arrows. In crude form, it's a strong poison. But a homeopathic preparation of this plant shares fame and popularity in the treatment of acute childhood conditions with *Belladonna,* a homeopathic remedy made from the poison of another powerful plant, deadly nightshade.

How would you feel if a homeopath prescribed you a remedy made from Bushmaster snake venom (*Lachesis,* one of the most popular and effective remedies)? I mean, how does anyone dare offer this stuff to people, let alone children? For years, homeopaths struggled with this issue. Although any homeopath knows how effective and safe homeopathic remedies are, telling people that they will be getting a remedy made of Wolf spider (*Tarentula)* or cancer cells (*Carcinosin)* has been always difficult.

On the other hand, there are remedies made from seemingly inert and harmless substances that, in their crude forms, couldn't possibly affect anything or anyone for better or for worse, let alone when given in a small dose. For example, the powerful and often prescribed remedy *Natrum muriaticum* is made out of common table salt. One of the cornerstones of constitutional treatment, *Calcarea carbonica* is made out of oyster shell. Essentially, it is carbonate of Lyme. *Lycopodium*, a remedy that treats literally thousands of symptoms, is made out of club moss seeds, which are so small that a large amount of them looks like flour. In Hahnemann's day, the seeds were considered biologically inert and used to cover pills of conventional medications.

Isn't it a total waste of time—even a deception—to offer patients table salt as a cure? And isn't it dangerous to offer patients snake venom or cancer cells? There is a simple way to reconcile the tremendous differences in the materials that go into the making of powerful homeopathic remedies. The key is in the method of preparation. Potentization is responsible for their therapeutic activity. Source materials may be poisons or inert substances. In either case, simple dilutions won't be effective at all. Only serial dilutions accompanied by vigorous shaking at each step do the trick. That's why homeopaths can have it both ways—safe and effective.

There's *no chance* that a homeopathic preparation made out of *any* substance will carry its infectious or poisonous qualities, as Hahnemann discovered a perfect method for extracting the curative qualities of various substances. So you can rest assured that your child won't get hurt by homeopathic *Carcinosin* or *Tarentula*.

The majority of classical homeopaths never give prescriptions below 12C, an attenuation at which the active substance in a remedy is exceedingly difficult to detect. The most popular attenuations for these products are 30C and 200C. Essentially, even if a small child ate all the pellets in the container at once, poisoning would be impossible.

For thousands of years, humanity has been using poisonous and potentially dangerous substances, in one form or another, for the purpose of healing. Like homeopathy, conventional medicine uses poisonous and biologically active substances. For example, manufacturers have long used whole cells of the pertussis bacteria to produce a vaccine for whooping cough. A new combination vaccine called DTaP (for diphtheria, tetanus, and pertussis) consists of only small, purified pieces of germs. A very old conventional drug, Digoxin, is a poison itself if given in large doses; in small doses it helps relieve chronic heart failure. But the same substance could kill if it were taken in its concentrated form. Of course, there are no live bacteria or viruses in any of these preparations. Their difference from homeopathic remedies is that they're significantly less diluted and not potentized at all. Unlike homeopathy, allopathic medicine is not familiar with turning inert substances into medications.

The ancient Romans had a proverb: *"Dosis facit venemon."* Translation: "It is the dose that makes the poison." As far as the safety of a homeopathic remedy is concerned, unnecessary repetition of doses is a much worse issue than the amount of the remedy taken at once. As you'll recall, homeopathic provings are conducted by giving healthy people repeated doses of a substance and monitoring the symptoms they develop.

Of course, a hypersensitive individual might respond poorly to a given remedy. A homeopath would appreciate this fact and make necessary adjustments to accommodate the sensitivity of the patient.

Homeopathic Aggravation

Many of those interested in homeopathy have heard about the aggravation, or "healing crisis," and are concerned that the remedies their friends, family and children are using could trigger one. What exactly is aggravation? Aggravation is a temporary reaction to the remedy. Usually, it lasts between a few minutes in acute conditions to a few days in chronic conditions. During an aggravation, symptoms of a past illness or of a current acute illness emerge and intensify. This phenomenon is part of the healing process.

Aggravations don't happen all the time, yet an aggravation is usually a clear indication of a correctly prescribed remedy. Symptoms initially worsen and then quickly go away, never to return. In cases when the aggravation is uncomfortably strong, which happens more frequently in constitutional than acute treatment, the best antidotes are conventional drugs because they work in a manner opposite to homeopathy: suppression.

You don't need to worry about this phenomenon when treating simple acute conditions with remedies in homeopathic concentration 30C. In over twenty years of practice, I can recall only two or three cases when an aggravation was so serious that it required some kind of suppression. All you need to do to prevent aggravations from happening is not repeat the remedy that prompted the aggravation for as long as the symptoms are improving.

There are two populations for whom it is always a good idea to consult professional homeopaths rather than home medicating: pregnant women and infants. In later sections of this book, you'll find possible solutions for a few self-limiting ailments for people in these two groups. To be safe, always consult with your primary care physician to make sure no potentially serious problems are hiding behind a seemingly benign symptom. Appropriately prescribed homeopathic remedies absolutely improve the course of pregnancy and the process of childbirth.

Infants and toddlers tolerate homeopathy perfectly well. The trouble is that they don't speak and so a layperson might not be able to figure out what remedy is indicated, whereas an experienced homeopath usually can make an accurate determination.

Administration and Storage of Homeopathic Remedies

Modern homeopathic remedies are usually sold packaged in sophisticated, easy-to-use dispensing systems. In administering the pellets, the main principles to follow are not to touch the pills and not to give too many of them to the recipient at the same time. Instructions on the container suggest giving three to five pellets per dose. You are actually welcome to give one or up to ten. Experience has shown that any number of pellets in this range is OK. Rely on what seems to be reasonable to you. A homeopath usually dispenses one pellet of 30C or a higher potency (for instance, 200C or 1M).

Remedies should be taken at least thirty minutes before a meal, and no sooner than thirty minutes after meal. It is preferable to dissolve pellets under the tongue. But there's evidence that swallowing a homeopathic remedy in this form also works fine.

Some people prefer taking liquid remedies. Tinctures are widely available. In the case of the administration of the liquid medication, you should give a few drops in a small amount of distilled water. You may also use the *plussing method,* described in the next section of this chapter, to prepare your own liquid dilutions.

Containers holding remedies should be stored in a dry dark place away from strong odors and electromagnetic radiation. Our times present new technological challenges, such as going through an X-ray machine at the airport. A curious homeopath exposed his homeopathic kit to this procedure forty times in a row to determine what kind of impact it would have. His remedies still worked fine afterward. But if you feel concerned, it can't hurt to show your remedies to security personnel and ask permission to bypass the screening. I've never yet met an airport screener who was unfamiliar with homeopathic remedies. (Maybe we should ask them to teach conventional physicians?)

The Plussing Method: How to Prepare Liquid Remedies

I always tell patients new to homeopathy, "If you thought what you heard so far seemed crazy, wait until I teach you how to dilute remedies."

In cases when you need to administer a remedy in a liquid form, perhaps because a small child or at times an older adult is reluctant to swallow a pellet, you can place a pellet in a small (half a liter or less) bottle of spring water. Make sure that you pour out approximately a third of the water from the bottle before adding the pill. Close the lid, wait for five minutes, and then shake the bottle vigorously eight to twelve times by hitting it against a book or the palm of your hand. Then give a person one teaspoon of the water. Close the lid and store the bottle at room temperature. It will remain good for two days. Each time you need to administer another dose, just shake the bottle again and give one teaspoon of the water again. There's no need to add more pellets.

This method is called *plussing*. It was developed by Hahnemann, and is described in paragraph 248 of his main work, *Organon of the Medical Art*. Many homeopaths like plussing and recommend using it for acute conditions, and even some chronic ones. The beauty of plussing is that you increase the potency of the remedy just a little bit each time you perform a succussion. This gives the remedy an additional "kick."

Plussing is useful for cases in which you notice that the initial dose of the remedy did the job effectively, but then the recipient got worse again. That means the person needs another dose of the same remedy. In such situations, plussing works very well. Repeating so-called dry remedies (meaning just pellets) is OK, too.

I started practicing homeopathy back in the day when there were no plastic bottles of spring water, or at least not in Russia. I used to recommend taking a third of a glass of distilled water or cooled boiled water, adding a pellet, covering the glass with a saucer, waiting for about five minutes, and then stirring it vigorously for twenty seconds. The results were exactly the same.

This method is reminiscent of Korsakov's dilution technique. But, of course, if anyone borrowed from someone else's idea, it was Korsakov using the method proposed by Hahnemann. Here's an example of how the plussing method taken to the extreme of Korsakoff's approach works.

In my days at Columbia University Medical Center, I was friendly with a professor in the field of molecular biology. He was originally from Ukraine where homeopathy is very popular. One day, he told me about his son having a severe case of acute sore throat. I offered him my services. I went over to his house with a few homeopathic remedies I'd brought from Russia. Very quickly I realized that my friend's ten-year-old son Sammy was presenting a typical picture of *Belladonna*. His throat was extremely sore, he had a high fever, his pupils were enlarged, and he looked confused.

Because I didn't have many pellets left, I suggested doing the following. They were to perform step one of the plussing method in the glass, and give Sammy a teaspoon of the solution. Then they were to pour out all of the water, put in fresh distilled water, stir it, and give the dose again if Sammy began to feel worse. Each time Sammy needed a new dose, the water had to be poured out and new water poured in without adding any more of the remedy.

It worked beautifully. Sammy felt better after the first dose, then in a few hours his fever went up and he was given a teaspoon of water that was added in the glass and stirred after the original solution was poured out. After the second dose the effect lasted even longer. The procedure had to be repeated only one more time.

Since then, I've prescribed homeopathy for practically all the members of the professor's family, including some grandchildren and a great-grandmother, with great success. I'm not asking you to go to such an extreme, but certainly the plussing method has its place in homeopathy.

Is It OK to Combine Remedies with Conventional Drugs?

There's an old joke that reminds me of how many people feel about homeopathy and conventional medicine. It goes something like this. A man gets stranded on an island. Fifteen years later, a cruise ship rescues him. Before leaving the island, the man offers the captain a tour. The captain is surprised to see two large huts standing opposite each other. The man explains, "This one is the shrine I go to, and that one is the shrine *I don't go to.*"

Although a few people in our culture use homeopathy or conventional medicine exclusively, in reality the majority of people combine them. If homeopathy or allopathic medicine is the "shrine" your family generally visits, and now you're considering visiting the other one, you need to be able to answer one of the following questions before you receive treatment.

- "If I am taking conventional drugs can I also take homeopathy?"
- "If I am taking homeopathy can I also take conventional drugs?"

Your safety or a family member's safety is obviously the main objective of any treatment strategy. Everything else comes second. But let's put one idea on the table from the beginning of this discussion. For better or worse, allopathic physicians provide more than 90 percent of the medical assistance that people receive in the modern, so-called civilized world. But M.D.s know extremely little about homeopathy. Their personal attitudes impact your care.

You, as a patient or parent/family member of the patient, wish to receive the best holistic care possible, and possibly you're upset that your physician doesn't know about homeopathy. If so, what can you do?

Should you stop seeing the conventional doctor? No. But if and when there's a window of opportunity for you to try a homeopathic solution, I suggest that you seize it. You can always fall back on conventional medicine. A rational combination of the two medical approaches would be ideal for pediatric, as well as adult health care.

Millions of people are alive today due to the existence of sterile surgical techniques, blood tests, magnetic resonance imaging, and rationally used antibiotics. The list of allopathic medicine's tremendous gifts is long. But, in an ideal world, whenever there was a need we'd first apply homeopathy, trying to resolve both acute and chronic conditions by strengthening our natural defense mechanisms. Upon occasion, we'd also turn to surgery. The use of heroic allopathic measures, including antibiotics, would be reserved only for those patients whose defense mechanisms couldn't overcome their illnesses without outside help, situations when the measures were absolutely warranted.

In this ideal world, homeopaths and allopaths would work together for the good of humanity. The ultimate outcome would be a much stronger, healthier generation who suffered fewer chronic illnesses, less mental illness, and engaged in less crime. Unfortunately, this kind of teamwork rarely exists today. Since the ideal is still a dream, how do you navigate the course to your and your children's total health?

Four Guidelines for Coordinating Your Health Care

It's important to find a doctor who'll be able to coordinate how various treatment modalities play out together, a health care "quarterback." Locating such a person may not be an easy task. It is much easier in major cities where there are usually integrative health care centers in which conventional providers who are complementary and alternative medicine (CAM)-friendly work hand in hand with homeopaths, acupuncturists, and other types of "alternative" practitioners. If you cannot find a place like that, the next best option is to ask if your pediatrician or family physician is open to CAM. Even better, seek a primary care physician who practices homeopathy.

Unfortunately, you may wind up feeling that you need to handle the coordination of treatment on your own. In that case, here are four guidelines you need to follow.

Guideline 1: Regardless of how incorrect and potentially damaging you believe the current treatment regimen is, *please do not discontinue conventional medications without professional medical advice.* You need to be clear on this point. A sudden cessation of medications may put a significant stress on your system—one so significant, in fact, that your condition may become much worse than before.

I cannot begin to tell you how often homeopaths have to face the following dilemma. The patient have "tried everything" and come to the homeopath as a last resort, hoping for a miracle. Now they immediately want all the medications stopped, either because the drugs aren't working or there are side effects. Even as I was writing this chapter, I had to deal with a situation where a couple were so excited by the improvement they saw after their son took a homeopathic remedy that they suddenly took him off his prescription drugs. Predictably, their son wound up getting sicker and they panicked.

Please understand that the only objective professional homeopaths have is to improve your, your family members and your children's health. And we need to do it in a safe way. If we rush the situation, the patient, who is already weak, may experience more damage.

The danger of suddenly discontinuing medication exists whether or not you subsequently receive homeopathy.

Guideline 2: Do not begin homeopathic treatment and allopathic treatment at the same time. With rare exceptions, use only one of these modalities at a time. If your child has chronic ear infections, for example, and currently is showing all the signs of a severe infection, it's a good idea to let your child undergo a full course of antibiotics first, and *then* to go see a homeopath. The homeopath can help you to cure the chronic problem that is causing repeated ear infections. Combining antibiotics with homeopathy wouldn't make sense, as these two approaches work in opposite directions. The former suppresses symptoms to achieve relief, whereas the latter helps express symptoms in order to cure them. Furthermore, if changes *do* occur while you're using both approaches simultaneously, you won't know to what to attribute them.

Of course, it's always your decision which way to go. For another condition, you might decide to ask a homeopath to treat you or your child first before trying a conventional medication. The important part is not to procrastinate in making a decision, because a delay may cause damage to your health. The same holds true for any condition in which you have to face a choice between homeopathic or allopathic treatment. Be proactive.

Good news. In acute situations, *correctly* prescribed homeopathic remedies work swiftly—usually right away. Therefore, you won't be in doubt for long about the results of your decision. But, in some cases, it can take a few tries to narrow in on the right remedy, called in homeopathy the simillimum (translated loosely from Latin it means the remedy most likely to restore health). So please don't wait until the very last moment! I often hear statements like this one. (The conversation happened at the end of July.) "Doc, we waited for so long and finally decided to start our son on Ritalin. Now we absolutely have to get results by the end of August, so you have three weeks to try." An impossible proposition!

Make up your mind if you want to use homeopathy, then determine your window of opportunity, and if it's too short at the moment, use whatever conventional method you need to in the meantime, and then come to the homeopath at the beginning of the next window of opportunity. Or, if there isn't a window, do what's suggested below.

Guideline 3: If you or your child have already been taking conventional medication for a few months, homeopathic treatment may safely be added. Your major defense mechanisms will have already adapted to the combination of stresses caused by the illness and the medication.

As I indicated in Guideline 1, your need to keep taking the conventional medications. Finding the right remedy for a person who's been receiving suppressive allopathic medications is difficult. But as homeopathy begins to work, the improvement will be obvious to the allopathic physician, and *then* discontinuation of the medication is possible. More and more allopathic physicians accept the fact that a large number of patients including children receive help from CAM providers. Professional dialogues are developing.

Guideline 4: If you are receiving homeopathic treatment, all new symptoms and conditions should be managed with the participation of your attending homeopath. Symptoms may only be evidence of a brief healing crisis, which from a homeopath's perspective shows the healing process is on track.

Before you do anything else—even apply a cream, give an aspirin, or use an inhaler—contact your homeopath—*right away.* Jumping the gun and rushing into a course of suppressive treatment can have disastrous consequences. We don't want to interfere with nature. I'll give you an example of what can happen.

Years ago, I treated Linda, a beautiful ten-month-old angel. Almost since her birth, Linda had an ear infection that required numerous courses of antibiotics. She went on to develop severe asthma attacks that required frequent visits to the ER. As her pediatrician knew about homeopathy, he suggested that her parents see whether or not I could help. The parents called to make an appointment while Linda was finishing a course of prednisone. We met a week after this hormone therapy was finished.

Linda's illness was severe and had frequent exacerbations, but she was a happy, personable child. Her emotional level was intact. Put together, these signs indicated that she was fighting her illness. For all the purposes of my evaluation, Linda was clearly at Level 2 health. Her symptoms and family history made the choice of remedy obvious. After only one dose, Linda began to improve and was illness-free in a few short weeks. The pediatrician was comfortable with the results. Linda didn't need further treatment.

At Linda's six-week follow-up I reinforced the same rules we're talking about here. Parents in my practice were told everything that you're reading. Nonetheless, a few months later, I received a phone call early in the morning from Linda's mother, who was frantic. The night before, her daughter had developed a fever of 101.3 Fahrenheit (38.5 Celsius) so Mom decided to give her some Tylenol. Although the fever went down due to the drug's suppressive action, in the morning Linda developed a cough and started to wheeze. Mom was extremely alarmed that Linda was having an asthma attack.

Because her daughter was suffering that day, I recommended to Linda's mother that she give Linda an asthma medication inhaler. By then there really was no other choice but to resort to a conventional drug. I told her to take Linda to see her pediatrician ASAP, and then, afterwards, to come see me. I immediately phoned the pediatrician, who also reached out to Linda's mother to ensure that in her state of panic she wouldn't forget to come see him that morning and receive additional instructions, if necessary. It is my belief, however, that the entire asthmatic episode might have been avoided if Linda's fever had been allowed to run its course with only a little help from homeopathy.

Of course, you should be prepared to go to the emergency room if the acute problem is severe enough to warrant it. Go to the ER if you can't get in touch with your homeopath in the course of ten to fifteen minutes. On the other hand, if your child has only a mild fever of 100 degrees.1 degrees, and is active and happy, you could wait a little bit longer. Same applies to an adult person, too. Use common sense. When in doubt, always seek professional help. Better safe than sorry!

Is It OK to Combine Remedies with Other Forms of Alternative Medicine?

As indicated above, it's better *not* to use more than one health care modality at a time, even when the treatments are natural, or biologically based, such as herbs and plant extracts. Theoretically, there's no valid distinction between the same person taking numerous conventional medications and taking numerous alternative medications, or any other combination of conventional and alternative product. It is always polypharmacy, which if you recall confuses the body's responses.

What about giving a child an additional homeopathic remedy (or more) while that child is been treated by a homeopath for a chronic problem? What harm can come from that? It is the same thing! Polypharmacy.

A good description of what can happen when various treatments are combined is contained in the following fable. A fool hires a lobster, a stork, and a donkey to move a carriage. He thinks the job will get done faster this way. The lobster will pull on the carriage from the river; the stork will pull from the sky; and the donkey from the ground. After hours of effort, however, the carriage doesn't move an inch. Why? Where does the fool's plan go awry? The laborers are pulling in opposite directions. Similarly, when several medications are taken, the body's functions work in opposition.

By the way, this principle of not mixing different forms of treatment can even be true for CAM modalities, such as osteopathy and craniosacral therapy, that don't involve the consumption of substances. I'll explain why in a moment. Let's take as an example what some parents do for their children as, naturally, most parents feel compelled to do the best they can for their children. Many assume more is better. Today, children often have busy schedules: a soccer game Sunday morning, ballet class Sunday afternoon, martial arts Monday and Thursday, cheerleading training Tuesday, piano and violin lessons on alternating Wednesdays, spinning class Friday night, and Japanese calligraphy Saturday. How's that for a happy childhood?

I've met many children whose parents regularly take them to see practitioners of Chinese medicine, Ayurveda, craniosacral therapy, osteopathy, and so on. The schedule offered by many so-called holistic specialists is similarly hectic. Their aim is to "chelate heavy metals" or "boost the immune system." Such children get caught up in a vicious cycle of being overtreated and overprescribed alternative medicines. Yet they don't get better. The popular premise called *synergism,* the concept that dissimilar modalities applied together are mutually supporting, is obviously wrong. More is *not* better.

To illustrate this concept, let me tell you how the parents of two autistic children who are my patients underwent a highly educational experience. For years they'd combined a variety of CAM approaches. After homeopathic treatment, the children improved somewhat, but not to a spectacular extent. Then, due to financial difficulties, the parents had to stop bringing them to all the care providers except for the homeopath. Surprisingly, the children started to improve at a much faster rate. This aptly illustrates my point: Each CAM modality can bring about significant improvement. Still it's better to utilize them judiciously, not necessarily at once.

By the way, when I had a very active full time homeopathic practice, many of the children I met had never had milk, bread, or candy. In fact, there was no real food in their lives anymore. The same was frequently true for their parents, too. Instead, their meals contained "proteins," "fats," "carbohydrates," and "supplements." Sound like a nightmare already? It is!

Why don't we stop and think about nutrition for a second. If adults or children have Level 1 health, they don't need vitamin and mineral supplements, and don't have to avoid eating regular foodstuffs. Yes, you and your children need to eat a balanced diet. Certainly, buying organic produce and products is a good idea, if you can afford them. Eating organic prevents chemicals and hormones from being introduced into our bodies. But only people with compromised health need to make *temporary* adjustments in their diets, such as eliminating wheat or dairy to control their allergic responses.

What about people with acute illnesses? Isn't it better to "hit" the immune system with a powerful "booster," such as an herb? Actually, it isn't necessary for those with Level 1 health. They only need gentle "reminders" of what their bodies naturally know to do. A homeopathic remedy is fine for this purpose.

People with Level 2 and Level 3 health do remarkably well on homeopathic treatments when they are faced with acute ailments. Of course, some people feel the need to introduce herbs into the mix at these times, and this is fine—especially when someone doesn't really know what remarkable results can be achieved by using homeopathy. Perhaps they've just read about it. While you're learning about homeopathy, try to use as few herbal supplements as you possibly can. Less is more with any treatment approach.

I was pleasantly surprised to learn that cranial therapists and osteopathic physicians ask their patients not to combine other CAM modalities with what they're doing. I've had personal experiences with Ayurvedic, Tibetan, and Chinese physicians, and most also suggest not combining modalities. There are two main reasons. First, we don't really know how various modalities interact with each other. All of them, including homeopathy, are built on the belief that illness and cure happen on an energetic plane. The influence each of these modalities has on the human energy system is very subtle. If there is a chance they'll interfere with each other, the consequences are unpredictable.

Secondly, if we combine modalities, how can we understand what did or didn't work, or what caused harm if the condition worsens? Allopathic medicine works on a concrete, physical level. That's why homeopathy may be superimposed on allopathic drugs without causing the kind of problems just described for CAM modalities.

Patients don't need to go at the same time to every single health professional that they can find. But if one is suffering from a chronic illness for which they are seeking homeopathic treatment, an informed decision should be made of what other therapies are absolutely necessary to keep doing—steps such as continuing a regimen of herbal medications the patient is already on—and what steps can wait.

If a person has been on the same CAM treatment regimen for a few months and they decide to see whether homeopathy can make a positive difference, adding a remedy to an already established therapy presents less of a problem than it would otherwise. Patient's body has probably stabilized its functions by now.

Of course, there are exceptions.

It is not uncommon for individuals receiving treatment for chronic conditions to develop acute ailments, such as colds and flu. In fact, acute illnesses that occur during ongoing constitutional treatment can be signs that the person's overall level of health is improving. But how should you handle an acute illness? Can you take a homeopathic remedy, or would that nullify the ongoing treatment? Can you use herbs? The best thing to do is to consult with your treating homeopath.

If the illness is a *true* acute illness, meaning that a patient has developed new, uncharacteristic symptoms in the midst of an ongoing illness, taking a new homeopathic remedy may or may not be indicated. Speak to your homeopath about it to be certain.

The rule of thumb is that herbal supplements are safe in such instances. They don't suppress the body's innate healing processes, nor do they interfere with homeopathy. Like herbs, Bach remedies are safe to use, as these formulas are made from flowers. Aromatherapy oils are very safe, so long as they're not ingested. Just be careful using eucalyptus, clove, mint, and peppermint oils around a person who is receiving homeopathic treatment. These oils may antidote, or nullify, the effect of homeopathy.

There's a potential complication, too. Symptoms that seem to be acute might actually be a part of the healing process initiated by homeopathy. According to Hering's Law, if a patient has ever had a similar symptom picture in the past, those symptoms may now be reemerging. If so, the situation becomes more complicated. Your homeopath *must* be involved in the decision-making process.

CHAPTER FOUR

Myths, Controversies, and Confusion

> *"I think that there is incredible prejudice about witches while there is no prejudice about wizards. Words are very important, and I'm really into destroying myths."*
> —YOKO ONO

Over the years, much confusion has arisen about the nature of homeopathy. Skeptics continue to attack its theoretical underpinnings. All sorts of unconventional therapies have been lumped together under a single banner, even though many have little to do with the basic principles that define the classical homeopathic approach. Here, we'll tackle the skeptics' claims head on, and sort through the various healing methods that appear more or less homeopathic.

Let's begin with six familiar misconceptions.

Six Myths about Homeopathy

An enormous amount of commentary about homeopathy is floating around in books by popular authors and on the internet. Some comes from homeopathic sources. Some comes from those who oppose homeopathy. What makes this flood of information so difficult for a layperson to handle is that the information is often contradictory and it is confusing. If you've been doing research, chances are good that you've encountered the same handful of misconceptions patients usually ask homeopaths to explain.

Myth 1: "Homeopathy Is a Placebo"

There's a legend that homeopathy is a placebo because it has no side effects, and because remedies are delivered to patients on nonactive sugar pellets.[1] But homeopaths know that correctly prescribed remedies for chronic conditions frequently cause an initial, sometimes significant worsening of the condition—an *aggravation*. Hahnemann and every homeopath since him have observed this effect. If even the most highly diluted homeopathic remedies are taken too frequently, they result in provings. Healthy, sensitive individuals develop symptoms commensurate with the remedy's picture.

If homeopathic remedies were placebos, aggravations simply wouldn't occur. This effect shows that remedies are active substances, even though they're highly diluted. But don't confuse an aggravation with a side effect. It's a healing response that quickly passes. It shows that the right remedy was taken. If the wrong remedy is consumed, no effects result.

As for the sugar pellets, remedies don't only come in this form. They can be delivered in the form of tinctures, ointments, tablets, gels, and lotions, too. Please don't confuse the means of delivery with the remedy itself.

By the way, studies show that the placebo effect occurs with every treatment modality. Did you know that even surgery has a high rate of placebo effect? Don't take my word for it. A 1994 article by A.G. Johnson published in one of the world's most prestigious medical journals, *The Lancet,* illustrates how.[2]

Research has also shown that the positive results of placebos tend to be short-lived. By contrast, homeopathic treatment leaves patients symptom-free for years.

Homeopathy is not a "fake." There's plenty of scientific evidence that it works. Hahnemann's scientific curiosity led him to reject the conventional harmful practices of his own day, much as this book is encouraging you to reject the harmful conventional practices of our day, such as the overuse of antibiotics. Hahnemann conducted numerous experiments and a thorough search of the professional literature, and these resulted in the discovery of the basic principles of homeopathy. He integrated every progressive discovery of the era, including the discovery of microbes, into his theory. Other scientists largely ignored microbes until Louis Pasteur did his work a few years later.

The nature of homeopathic dilutions remains controversial for conservative allopathic scientists and physicians. Nobody, including homeopaths, likes the fact that to date we can't really understand how and why high dilutions work in the human body. We just can't explain this phenomenon yet. Some remarkable pieces of research suggest that the serial process of dilution and succussion results in the formation of crystalline structures in water that possibly could be the carriers of biological information. But these studies are preliminary. They provide no definitive answer to the mechanism by which ultramolecular homeopathic dilutions produce their healing effect.

In reality, lots of effective medications and therapies don't have well-established mechanisms of action. Clinical results therefore constitute the best jury. And there the verdict is clear: well-designed clinical studies prove homeopathy different from placebo.

At the time of this writing, two meta-analyses of the clinical effects of homeopathy have been published: the first in the *British Medical Journal* (1991), and the second in *The Lancet* (1997). Meta-analysis is research in which data from multiple independent studies on the same subject are pulled together and evaluated collectively. I'm going to get a little bit more technical here to satisfy our most inquisitive readers.

The *British Medical Journal* review assessed 107 controlled trials in ninety-six published reports. Overall, of the 105 trials with interpretable results, eighty-one trials indicated positive results versus twenty-four trials in which no positive effects of homeopathy were found. In studies judged to have better research designs, fifteen trials showed positive results, whereas in seven trials no positive results could be detected. This is significant evidence in favor of homeopathy.[3]

The review in *The Lancet* assessed 186 double blind and/or randomized trials. Eighty-nine of these publications had adequate data for meta-analysis. The combined odds ratio was 2.45 in favor of homeopathy. The odds ratio for the twenty-six good quality studies was 1.66, and when it was corrected for estimated publication bias (meaning corrected for researchers intent on showing positive results) the ratio remained about the same (1.78). These results are also very significantly in favor of homeopathy's clinical effectiveness.[4]

In other words, homeopathy helps people feel better, which is where it counts.

Nineteenth-century British Prime Minister Benjamin Disraeli once said: "There are three kinds of lies: lies, damned lies, and statistics." He had a point. Unfortunately, if someone has his mind set on disproving a scientific claim, or for that matter proving a claim, it is easy to manipulate data in support of that goal. Intentionally, or perhaps unintentionally, researchers have often stacked the deck against homeopathy in the way they design their research protocols. The authors of these studies almost religiously follow the notorious principle: If you ask a silly question, you'll get a silly answer.

Almost every time a study on homeopathy has been designed and carried out by experienced homeopaths, however, its results have been promising. I know that this statement doesn't come as a surprise. Naturally, one would expect reliable studies on gynecology to be designed by gynecologists, and reliable studies on psychiatry to be designed by psychiatrists, and so on. Please bear these observations in mind each time you do your own literature search and read scientific papers about homeopathy.

A prominent researcher, Daniel Eskinazi, D.D.S., Ph.D., published an interesting paper, entitled "Homeopathy Re-revisited,"[5] in the prestigious medical journal *Archives of Internal Medicine* (1999). In it, he demonstrated that if the tenets of homeopathy are restated in modern biomedical parlance, they not only make a lot of sense, they're also fully supported by data from conventional medical textbooks and research.

Myth 2: "You Have to Believe in Homeopathy for It to Work"

This statement presumes that homeopathy is a placebo, and any positive results it produces should be attributed to the power of suggestion. Not so! Every homeopath has handled many cases of skeptical patients coming in prejudiced against homeopathy. They come under the pressure of a spouse or a parent. Homeopathy still works. Believing in it isn't really necessary. It's hard to imagine that merely our best intentions would have been so consistently helpful in curing serious diseases for over 200 years.

Myth 3: "Homeopathy Is a Cult That's 'Frozen' in the Nineteenth Century"

From functioning as an advanced, scientifically sound branch of medicine during the nineteenth century and early twentieth century, homeopathy was marginalized in America to something similar to a cult during the second half of the twentieth century. This wasn't the case elsewhere in the world, for instance in England, France, Germany, India, and Russia. Due to the rivalry in the United States between those who practice conventional medicine and homeopathy, the resources of modern science weren't as readily available to homeopaths as to allopaths. There weren't any homeopathic institutions. Medical schools, industry, and the government allocated their resources to a different set of interests.

The problem was compounded by the fact that homeopathic remedies have been in the public domain for so long. Pharmaceutical companies fund a great deal of medical research in this country and elsewhere. But most don't consider the research and development of nonproprietary medications, such as homeopathic remedies, a good financial investment, as remedies cannot be patented and exclusively sold.

One day soon, I hope we will see the reemergence of full-time homeopathic schools and homeopathic research laboratories. In the meantime, we are blessed with the support of the Samueli Institute for Information Biology, headed by prominent scientist Wayne B. Jonas, M.D. This organization sponsors basic scientific and clinical research on homeopathy and energy medicine. Jonas is a former director of the

Office of Alternative Medicine for the National Institutes of Health (NIH) and former Director of the Medical Research Fellowship at the Walter Reed Army Institute of Research.

All around the world, scientists like Jonas are conducting research on homeopathy. Two other prominent American researchers are Iris Bell, M.D., Ph.D., and Jennifer Jacobs, M.D. Despite the lack of funds for biomedical research, homeopathic theory and practice have been developing in leaps and bounds. In the last two decades, homeopaths have developed and sharpened new tools for the analysis of patients. For example, homeopaths all use sophisticated homeopathic software now that allows us to cross-reference important symptoms and conduct effective literature searches in minutes. Certainly this type of analysis requires extensive training in classical homeopathy. A computer cannot find appropriate remedies by itself. But it is a great time saver.

The homeopathic community has been using new, in-depth approaches to case analysis. Practicing homeopaths spend many hours studying cases and literature. We host numerous national and international professional seminars and conferences. AIH has an annual meeting. The National Center for Homeopathy (NCH) has an annual meeting. The Liga Medicorum Homoeopathica Internationalis (LMHI), an international organization of homeopathic physicians, also conducts meetings annually. There are also many periodic homeopathic publications. Homeopathy is very much alive and advancing.

Although homeopathy went through a dark age of being denied a right to exist, those times are now over. Practitioners of homeopathy, as well as other CAM modalities, are allowed to treat patients and conduct research. Some conventional physicians still assert that homeopaths shouldn't be allowed to conduct research because homeopathy is a "fake." But the NIH is curious about alternative medicine. Research will do only one thing: help develop reliable homeopathic practice.

Myth 4: "Homeopathy Is Harmless No Matter What You Do"

It's dangerous to believe that homeopathy can be used as frequently as you wish and in any dose. The truth is that homeopathy *only* remains harmless *so long as you don't abuse it*. But if you follow the advice in this book and only take a single dose of one homeopathic remedy at a time, then, yes, homeopathy is safe.

Myth 5: "Mint 'Antidotes' the Effects of Homeopathy"

Old popular books on homeopathy contain the suggestion that mint counteracts, or neutralizes, the effects of remedies. It isn't accurate. What would be accurate is that taking a homeopathic remedy immediately after you've brushed your teeth with mint-containing toothpaste isn't a good idea. The pleasant cool feeling that mint and peppermint produce in the mouth is the result of the constriction of capillaries (small blood vessels). Homeopathy is administered under the tongue to ensure that the remedy gets into the bloodstream as soon as possible. Constricting the blood vessels right before taking the remedy isn't a good idea as it interferes with absorption.

Many homeopathic patients buy special "homeopathic" toothpaste. These actually contain several homeopathic remedies and might interfere with the progress of treatment. In case you still want to play it safe, there are many kinds of toothpaste without mint. But it's not important. You are welcome to eat mint candies, mint ice cream, and so on.

For some reason, various food items do antidote (counteract) certain remedies. Your homeopath will know what these are. Certain individuals are more sensitive than others, and thus it is easier to counteract remedies in such individuals.

In general, remedies are neutralized by allopathic medications; camphor (found in rubs like Tiger Balm and Wicks); strong electromagnetic fields (EMFs), such as those emanating from microwave ovens and plug-in alarm clocks; coffee; dental work; and some aromatherapy oils.

Myth 6: " Homeopathic Remedies Act Like Vaccines"

Superficially this statement seems accurate. After all, in both cases it seems as if a person is being given small quantities of a disease in order to avoid the disease. In reality, vaccination and homeopathy are based on *similar,* but not *identical* theories. Homeopathy follows the principle of similars, whereas the same vaccines are given to everyone.

Vaccination stimulates the immune system directly. This process results in the production of antibodies specific to a particular illness. Homeopathy works on a subtler, dynamic level and, most probably, activates all the body's major integrative systems.

Vaccines are tested on animals and are known to cause numerous adverse effects. Homeopathy is tested on humans (provings) and does not have side effects.

This myth leads us to the heart of a debate that's taken place for many years.

Is There Such a Thing as Homeopathic Prophylaxis?

Benjamin Franklin wrote, "An ounce of prevention is worth a pound of cure."[6]

All parents understand the wisdom of that expression. Measures designed to prevent disease are called *prophylaxis,* and date back to the most ancient of times. People have always wanted protection from the adversities of life, and they've always prayed for the health of their children. As soon as early humans recognized a divine influence, they started creating amulets, or tokens of divine protection. Some carried minerals, gems, and dried animal parts; some carried prayers engraved in stone or on precious metals; others enclosed prayers written on scrolls in leather pouches and other containers. These kinds of prophylaxis continue. Nowadays people frequently wear religious symbols around their necks, or they tie a red string around their wrist or another part of the body.

The majority of questions about prophylaxis are actually directed toward the prevention of infections. An infection, or an infectious disease, is often defined as a pathological state resulting from the invasion of the body by pathogenic microorganisms (bacteria or viruses). Yet let us rephrase this statement: Infection is a result of the *interaction* of the microorganism (a bacteria or virus) and the macroorganism (a human being). The important point is that a bug is not the same thing as an illness, although it is an important component in disease.

A number of publications have indicated that regular allopathic vaccines and aggressive schedules of their administration could be harmful to children. Thus, increasingly, parents are seeking so-called homeopathic vaccinations and prophylaxis.

Is there any validity to these practices? Is there such thing as *homeopathic* prophylaxis? Is there such a thing as *homeopathic* vaccination? There is no blanket answer. The truth can be found somewhere in the middle ground.

The situation is clear. To protect our children from infectious disease, we can kill the bugs, we can make our children stronger, or we can do both.

Killing the Bugs

We can destroy bacteria outside of the body. This is done using personal hygiene and sterilization techniques. We can also try to kill or at least weaken microbes that have invaded the body already. That's done with antibiotics. At the beginning of the twentieth century, when modern biomedical science was established, this approach was popular. It dramatically improved the outcome of surgery. It allowed us to combat infections, such as pneumonia and tuberculosis.

This approach worked well until we noticed that, on the one hand, bacteria were developing resistance to numerous antibiotics and, on the other hand, humans were developing allergic reactions and chronic infections. Furthermore, it turned out that in the process of killing the real enemy with our powerful antibiotics we winded up causing enormous collateral damage. We were killing friendly bacteria in the gut that we really need. Antibiotics also weaken our immune system; after all it is made from cells similar to bacteria. It causes confusion in the parts of the immune system responsible for recognizing the difference between what is "us" (our normal tissues and cells) and what is "foreign" (bacteria, viruses, and sick, deformed cells from within the body).

Making Children Stronger

Another preventive approach is to strengthen our children's natural defenses, so they can fight infections more effectively, and avoid becoming chronically ill or dying. Parents can participate by using homeopathy for first aid and treatment of mild acute conditions. Homeopaths can offer constitutional treatment to children whose bodies are weaker and more sensitive to the environment. These steps strengthen all of the body's integrative systems, which is the aim of this handbook.

Children also need:
- A stable, positive environment.
- Physical exercise.
- Appropriate rest.
- Adequate sleep.
- Good nutrition.
- Vitamin and mineral supplements (if necessary).

For homeopathy to help individual children become more resilient to disease, finding a remedy depends upon the *individual* characteristics of a *particular* child.

In the case of homeopathic prophylaxis, everything depends on identifying a *particular* disease in a *particular* population. This is something only a homeopath that sees large numbers of patients can do. It's a public health matter.

In 1801, Hahnemann attended a family with four children during a severe epidemic of scarlet fever. Three of the children contracted the illness. But the fourth and weakest child didn't! Hahnemann remembered that he'd just treated the boy for other problems with *Belladonna*. It was the only difference between him and his siblings. Soon after, Hahnemann attended a family with eight children. Three children had scarlet fever already. He gave *Belladonna* to the other five and they didn't get sick. Hahnemann began giving *Belladonna* to other children with scarlet fever. All were cured. Those who were treated prophylactically didn't get sick. Thus, homeopathic prophylaxis was discovered.

Now, despite this success, in later years *Belladonna* wasn't found effective for scarlet fever. A group of homeopathic physicians challenged

Hahnemann on this issue. By that time he'd clearly developed the concept of a *genus epidemicus,* the one remedy that corresponds to the picture of an epidemic illness in a particular population (people in a particular area at a particular time). Once you know the genus epidemicus, you can administer it to individuals within the population to prevent them from developing that illness. It's presumed that this remedy will be used for the duration of the threat.

For example, if there were flu in New York City in November, a homeopath working in New York might start seeing numerous children requiring *Gelsemium*. Their colleagues in New York and New Jersey might also begin to see a number of cases requiring *Gelsemium*. So we'd know that our genus epidemicus was probably *Gelsemium*. In this case, most people in the area could stay well by taking *Gelsemium* 12C every day for the duration of the epidemic.

Come December, we might start seeing a lot of cases that responded to another remedy, let's say *Arsenicum album*. As we begin to see more and more patients cured with *Arsenicum album*, we would realize that the genus epidemicus has changed. *Gelsemium* would no longer be the right remedy to take for prophylaxis.

That's how homeopathic prophylaxis works. It's like finding a group simillimum.

During the terrible flu epidemic of 1918 homeopaths identified three major genus epidemicus remedies. The death rate among people who received one of these remedies prophylactically or was treated with them was 1 percent. Several remedies had to be used because the illness migrated to different geographical regions of the country and infected different populations that were sensitive to different components of the illness.

As you can see, the best preventive homeopathic remedy can be selected only *after* an epidemic begins and homeopaths are able to prescribe the same remedy correctly to a number of people. We truly can't predict ahead of time. Nevertheless, the idea that there could be certain remedies for prevention of certain diseases remains popular.

To be clear: Homeopathic prophylaxis works only for as long as someone takes the *right* remedy. Usually homeopaths recommend taking lower potencies (12C or 30C) on a daily basis for the duration of an epidemic. In cases when people don't have any lead-time, administration of the remedy will cure most cases of the illness right away. Of course, there are always going to be some exceptions of people who require a different remedy. But the stronger a bug is, the more likely it is that the majority of people in the same region will require the same remedy at the same time.

Homeopathic Vaccination

Now we're ready to talk about the subject of *homeopathic vaccination*.

Conventional vaccination is a method directed at providing a permanent defense against an infection, one that doesn't require the daily use of medication. Ideally, one or a few applications of a vaccine would provide lifelong protection.

Vaccinations work in a specific way: by stimulating the immune system to develop antibodies to a particular infection. In the majority of cases, the effectiveness of vaccines can be measured by a test that measures titers of antibodies. If titers aren't high enough, it means that vaccine isn't effective. If titers decrease significantly, it means that the person needs a *booster*, another administration of the same vaccine.

It's fair to say that allopathic vaccines hurt a certain population of children. Not everyone is hurt, but some children are. It's also fair to say that vaccines have saved a lot of children. No one on this planet has small pox anymore. Go ahead and ask your pediatrician when the last time was that she saw a case of diphtheria—probably never. The same is true for polio. Those successes can be attributed to vaccinations.

Vaccinations played a crucial rule in saving lives during COVID-19 pandemic.

The website of the Center for Disease Control and Prevention (CDC) states:

In the first ten months that COVID-19 vaccines were available, they saved over 200,000 lives and prevented over 1.5 million hospitalizations in the United States. This is the purpose of these vaccines: to save lives and prevent severe disease. They can also reduce the risk of Long COVID.[7]

It certainly would be nice to be able to identify children and, later in life, adults who potentially could be hurt by vaccinations or even by a particular type of a vaccine. Then we could either treat them constitutionally and vaccinate, or not vaccinate them at all. We'd have a choice.

There are at least two questions that we need to answer in relation to this point.

1. Is it possible to prevent side effects of vaccinations with homeopathy?
2. Is it possible to vaccinate children (or adults for this matter) using homeopathic preparations of vaccines?

Most homeopaths field questions about the prevention of side effects. A lot of parents have heard about using *Thuja, Silicea,* or *Hypericum* for the "prophylaxis" of side effects from vaccinations. The belief is that if we gave every child let's say *Thuja* 200C before vaccination, it would protect all the children from negative side effects, while also allowing their immune systems to develop antibodies. Such a belief is simply false.

The same rumor applies to other remedies.

It would be more accurate to presume that children who constitutionally require one of the remedies listed above may be more prone to developing side effects from vaccinations. These children, and only these children, would potentially benefit from these remedies, because, as you know, we are looking for the simillimum, the one right remedy. There is no one-size-fits-all dosing in the classical homeopathic approach.

The best thing parents can do to prevent side effects from conventional vaccinations is to take their children for full homeopathic evaluations and constitutional treatment beforehand. Of course, figuring out what remedy is needed for a baby who can't talk, only consumes mother's milk, and has absolutely no symptoms is very tricky, if not impossible. But if the child is generally sensitive and has various persistent symptoms, such an assessment is possible. Appropriate homeopathic treatment may be helpful in warding off the side effects of vaccinations. It would be nice to be able to conduct such an assessment so early in a child's life, as we could then predict who needs special precautions or treatment.

Another consideration against the use of remedies to prevent side effects from conventional vaccines is that each time there's a vaccination visit to the doctor the child gets a few shots. Using the same remedy as often as conventional doctors give their shots isn't a good idea at all. It might cause a proving or otherwise derail the child's wellness. And it just contributes to the polypharmacy mixture. Homeopaths are familiar with the so-called confused cases that occur when patients receive multiple doses of homeopathic remedies. Treating these patients is a challenging proposition!

Yet another argument against this type of "prevention" is that there's absolutely no data on whether or not it is efficacious. Anecdotally, some homeopaths recommend it. Others don't. Based on what you know about the principles of homeopathy by now, I'm sure you can see that it probably doesn't make too much sense.

It's worth noting that some parents and medical professionals have questioned the efficacy, safety, and necessity of conventional childhood vaccines since immunization techniques were first conceived. Recently the term *vaccine-injured children* was used to describe the population of children today who show allergic and other negative reactions to different vaccines. In response to these concerns, homeopathic vaccination methods developed practically alongside conventional vaccination methods.

Beginning with Samuel Hahnemann, who introduced them, early homeopaths were interested in using nosodes to prevent infectious diseases. Constantine Hering later suggested the prophylactic use of *Lyssinum* (homeopathically prepared rabies) fifty years before Louis Pasteur's famous rabies vaccine. But he never used nosodes himself.

Later homeopaths suggested using specific nosodes for prophylaxis of specific diseases. For example, using *Anthracinum* for anthrax, *Pertussin* for whooping cough, and *Variolinum* for smallpox. If this attractive proposition worked, it would simplify the search for the simillimum. Rather than conducting a full interview and searching for the exact remedy, a homeopath would only need to identify the illness at hand and give out the corresponding nosode.

Nosodes were also suggested for use as "homeopathic vaccines." Today, many practitioners and parents have adopted this approach as an alternative to conventional vaccination. According to proponents, homeopathic vaccines induce the immune response and provide protection similar or even superior to conventional vaccines—without side effects. Certainly, homeopathic preparation are less expensive and don't contain additives, such as mercury, which conventional vaccines do.

I certainly wish things were so simple.

To date, the jury is out on the safety and efficacy of homeopathic vaccines. The idea is closer to allopathic medicine than homeopathy, which is always based on the individualization of treatment. But if something works well and causes no harm, it does not really matter if it is homeopathy, allopathic medicine, prayer, or acupuncture. So we only have to ask: Is there a sufficient amount of evidence that homeopathic vaccination is effective and harmless? The answer on both points is no.

The main reason we can't answer yes is that the number of well-designed studies on homeopathic vaccination is very small. As a matter of fact, the only well designed study was conducted on mice by Wayne Jonas, who published his finding in *Alternative Therapies in Health and Medicine* (1999).[8] In this study, 142 male mice were exposed to a deadly disease, tularemia. A standard vaccine protected them in 100 percent of cases. Nosodes averaged 22 percent. Of course, it is only one study, and other studies could produce better (or worse) results.

No one will conduct this type of placebo-controlled studies on humans, or even "side-by-side" studies of homeopathy vs. conventional vaccines. But there is some anecdotal evidence from the past. Most of this data was published in homeopathic journals and is difficult to access. For example, a group of authors from Brazil published an interesting paper in the *Journal of American Institute of Homeopathy*.[9] They reported that in 1974 during the outbreak of meningitis in Brazil, 18,640 patients were given the homeopathic nosode *Meningococcinum* as prophylaxis. There were only four cases of meningitis reported in this group. A control group of 6,340 people, who didn't receive any treatment, developed thirty-two cases. The efficacy seems to be obvious.

On the other hand, during the 1958 influenza epidemic in Great Britain, 1,100 subjects received homeopathic *Influenzinum* and 500 had no treatment. There was no difference between these two groups. In three different studies conducted in 1932, 1941, and 1946 by various researchers, children developed significant immune response to a homeopathic nosode *Diphtherinum*. The fact that three independent research groups reproduced the same protocol is significant, however it is only one study.

One of the most important reported features of conventional vaccination is that it provides long-term protection after just a few injections, called booster shots. A vocal proponent of homeopathic vaccination is Isaac Golden, a homeopath from Australia. He has published books on homeopathic vaccination and also wrote an interesting article for *Homeopathy Online,* an internet publication. According to his recommendations, children have to receive twenty-eight doses of nosodes during the first five years of life.

Golden's schedule is purely arbitrary. There's no particular reason to utilize this, or any other protocol. He reports that 10 percent of children experience some kind of "reaction" to the nosodes. Twenty-eight doses of various highly potentized homeopathic remedies may cause significant effects other than the alleged protection from the target illnesses. They actually may create additional long-term health problems that would be difficult to treat with homeopathy. Interestingly, Golden suggests using the nosodes again if an epidemic of one of the target illnesses begins. This means that there's no certainty that children are actually immunized after going through his elaborate protocol.

As you can see, the issue of homeopathic vaccination is complicated. Certainly, the clinical experience of 200 years demonstrates that genus epidemicus prescribing has always been a forte of homeopathy. It clearly shows impressive results when used according to the principles noted above. Constitutional treatment also clearly strengthens the defenses of our children and improves their level of health. Furthermore, children born to women who were treated with homeopathy during pregnancy are reported to be healthier. However, no controlled research studies on this subject are available.

Now you have sufficient information to draw your own conclusions.

What Homeopathy Is and What It Isn't

To state the obvious: Everyone prefers simple solutions. But the quest for a panacea, a miracle drug that could treat all illnesses at once, is doomed to failure. It doesn't exist. The next best thing would be one remedy for a particular illness. That's what conventional medicine is seeking. But this miracle doesn't exist either. We see this in the way individuals respond to the medications that are prescribed to them.

Happily, an effective remedy for one person does exist! By providing an individualized approach, classical homeopathy offers us this solution.

What Homeopathy Is

Classical homeopathy is a term coined to distinguish homeopathy practiced according to the original principles discovered by Hahnemann from everything else. More than 90 percent of American homeopaths practice classical homeopathy. This book is based on the classical homeopathic approach, which has three main features.

1. The principle of similars
2. Minimal dose
3. Single remedy

Pluralistic homeopathy is another form of homeopathy that's popular in France. Pluralists use frequent dosing and they alternate different remedies throughout the day. Unlike classical homeopathy, this approach is deeply rooted in pathology—changes that can be perceived—with a significant emphasis on concrete changes observed during the physical exam. The patient is kept busy taking medication. At times people are asked to take up to ten different remedies in different concentrations at different times of the day.

Certainly, classical homeopaths disapprove of these prescribing practices, although pluralists are known to get decent results. Most probably, the effect of multiple remedies and frequent dosing is suppressive. However, I know a few well-trained "pluralists" who actually use single remedies most of the time despite their background.

Regionally, homeopaths differ in regard to the potencies they use. The majority of North American homeopaths use centesimal dilutions (for example, 30C and 200C). Usually, the higher a dilution one uses, the less frequently one needs to take it. By contrast, homeopaths from Argentina and some other countries use decimal dilutions (for example, 3X and 6X). These preparations are taken a few times a day.

In many cases, modifications of homeopathy lead practitioners to deviate from the basic principles that make homeopathy most effective. Their so-called improvements and advances actually render these new methods non-homeopathic and ineffective. Essentially, these variations involve using homeopathic remedies in an allopathic manner. So far, the clinical results of these "innovative" methods haven't been as impressive as for classical homeopathy.

Interestingly, the future of allopathic medicine itself seems to lie in the direction of differential therapeutics, a term for utilizing more individualized treatment of patients, for instance for cancer. It's clear to everyone that different people's bodies respond with variations to the same medication. In prescribing conventional drugs, some doctors try to harness side effects to assist their patients' secondary complaints. For instance, if two patients have been diagnosed with the same disease, but one is lethargic and the other has insomnia, and there's a medication for the disease that in addition to its intended action also induces drowsiness, the doctor may give it to the insomniac patient. Why not make use of it?

Homeopathic Combination Remedies

The most prominent items in the homeopathic section of most health food stores are the so-called combination remedies. They are definitely bestsellers. These products seem to offer a simple and straightforward solution: one medication for one diagnosis. We can find combination remedies for almost anything that ails us, conditions ranging from teething and head colds to premenstrual syndrome and hemorrhoids. Combination remedies exist on the border of homeopathy and allopathic medicine because they are efficacious, like other homeopathic approaches, but they are prescribed for a condition and not for an individual. They're also examples of homeopathic polypharmacy. Most importantly, at times they provide very efficacious, temporary relief, but not a cure.

Are these remedies good? Some are useful for self-limiting conditions in strong individuals: Those with Level 1 or Level 2 health. The major homeopathic companies use combinations that have been tested for years and shown effective, but to reiterate, only for the *temporary* relief of self-limiting conditions, like the common cold or a bruise. Treating serious and or chronic conditions with combination remedies isn't a good idea.

The idea of combination remedies seems to be very simple. Two or more remedies known to relieve a particular symptom, or sometimes an illness, are combined in the same tablet. The expectation is that either the action of the combination will be synergistic (meaning the remedies will enhance each other), or that at least one of the remedies will be exactly what the patient needs.

Frederick Humphreys, M.D., a homeopath who got kicked out of the AIH and the New York State Homeopathic Medical Society for using them, introduced combination remedies into practice in 1885. He created them to reconcile the homeopathic and allopathic approaches, an impossible proposition. He hoped that there would be specific remedies for certain illnesses. But the premise is wrong. In homeopathy, we treat the whole person. We base prescriptions on the indicators that make people different from one another, rather than the symptoms that make everyone the same. What combination remedies do instead is to offer a quick fix to the public.

Setting that erroneous notion aside, we also know that any type of polypharmacy is considered to be highly undesirable in both allopathic and allopathic medicine. Do you recall the story about the lobster, stork, and donkey pulling in different directions?

Another common mistake is calling a remedy homeopathic just because it was diluted and potentized. A remedy is actually considered homeopathic only because of the manner in which it is being used. In order to be used homeopathically, the substances don't have to be diluted or shaken. Early homeopaths used drops of pure tinctures. The main feature of homeopathy is the application of medicinal substances according to the principle of similars.

Hahnemann clearly said in his main work *Organon of the Medical Art*: "In no case of cure is it necessary to employ more than a single simple medicinal substance at one time with patient."[10]

Some combination remedies are effective for *temporary* relief of symptoms. There are impressive combination remedies that palliate vertigo, inflammation, and teething. If you're going to use combination remedies, please remember that use should be limited and it might be suppressive. Any claim that a company has found an "easy solution" is not accurate at all. Real healing requires an understanding of individual traits.

An important consideration is whether or not combination remedies can damage you. If a person has Level 1 or Level 2 health, most probably you or your child will either benefit from a short course of, let's say, a teething combination, or that nothing at all will happen. A combination remedy might harm a child or an adult who is weaker and more sensitive.

As a general rule of thumb, don't use combination remedies if you are under the care of a professional homeopath. These preparations, as well as other medications, might interfere with the progress of constitutional treatment.

Cell Salts (Tissue Salts)

Cell salts have been presented to consumers as a different type of medicine than homeopathy, although in truth they are homeopathic preparations. They are sold in many health food stores, sometimes without a detailed description of what they are made from. Some parents believe that if they give cell salts to their children they can speed up their kids' growth, cure their sinus problems and other chronic infections, and help them overcome sleep disorders. Bottom line, cell salts are marketed as medicine in their own right, but they are an extension of homeopathy. They are only effective medicine, however, if they're prescribed by a homeopath who's utilizing the principle of similars. A parent should not prescribe cell salts for their own children.

Cell salts are made from some of the chemical elements found inside the cells of the human body. They are also found elsewhere in nature. German physician Wilhelm Schuessler introduced them in 1873. He erroneously thought he had found a new principle of cure. But he denied any connection with homeopathy. His original article published in German went unnoticed until a small book by Constantine Hering entitled *Twelve Tissue Remedies* was published in May 1873. Then, Schuessler witnessed twenty-five editions of his book get printed before his death in 1898. In the later editions, he denied any connection between his method and homeopathy. He insisted that his method was based only on the biochemistry of the human cell.

Scheussler's theory was based on the idea that the structure and vitality of the organs of the human body are dependent upon certain quantities of minerals present in human cells. His theory had no experimental basis. Cell salts are homeopathically prepared, usually in potencies of 3X, 6X, 12X, and 30X. He used most of the salts in 6X, and only a few at 12X. His biochemical theory also talks about the content of the cell salts in various homeopathic remedies. What makes cell salts unique is they are prepared all the way by trituration. As you may recall, trituration is the process Hahnemann devised to convert insoluble materials into a form that could be introduced into the core process of dilution and succussion. In classical homeopathy, triturations are only used for the first three steps of the attenuation process.

Schuessler suggested the use of twelve preparations. Modern homeopathic companies sell fourteen. The two additional ones are combinations. One of them is called Bioplasma. It contains all twelve cell salts: nine in 3X, and the remaining three in 6X. Another combination is called Biochemic Phosphates. It contains only the five salts that contain phosphates. According to the proponents of this combination, it's supposed to be good for the nervous system. All the remedies in this combination are 3X.

Schuessler subscribed to the individualization of treatment, and actually there is a short cell salt repertory available in various editions of his work, as well as in books on the methodology of cell salt treatment. All twelve cell salt remedies are also used as regular homeopathic preparations in the practice of classical homeopathy. But classical homeopaths do not subscribe to Scheussler's biochemical theory. We simply happen to use preparations made from the same materials because most of them existed *before* Schuessler. For example, *Calcarea salts* and *Silicea* are homeopathic remedies first described by Hahnemann. Although, slow acting, cell salts shouldn't be used without control or appropriate advice from trained homeopaths. The prophylactic use of cell salts is of questionable value both from the therapeutic and safety points of view.

What Homeopathy Isn't

Homeopathy is everything that uses the principle of similars. Everything else is *not* homeopathy. Methods described in this section aren't necessarily "bad" practices. Some, such as herbal medicines, are quite efficacious. They just aren't homeopathy. Frequently, medical treatment is mysterious. While mystery may be appealing to some, my view is that having a clear understanding of what is going on or *not* going on during any treatment is important for ensuring safety.

Herbal Medicine

A large number of people come to my office with the mistaken belief that homeopathy and herbal medicine are the same. In fact, they are like apples and oranges. Homeopathic remedies are potentized, and must be administered one at the time. By contrast, herbs are neither diluted nor succussed, and herbal medicines are often administered several at a time. Additionally, homeopathic remedies are made from various natural substances, which include, but are not limited to herbs.

Bach Flower Remedies

Many people considered the Bach Flower Remedies to be part of the field of homeopathy. They are not. Dr. Edward Bach (pronounced "Batch") started his career as a bacteriologist and pathologist at the London Homeopathic Hospital. Homeopathy became his main interest, and in 1926 he coauthored a book on homeopathy. He was also interested in plants. In 1930, he left London and went to the countryside to investigate the healing power of flowers. He ultimately developed thirty-eight flower essences. Although frequently referred to as homeopathic, these interesting and effective remedies are not homeopathic in the way they are prepared, nor in the way they are used for treatment.

Bach rejected the cornerstone principle of similars. He believed in natural beauty, and that good replacing evil would lead to "true healing." In his book *Heal Thyself,* he suggested that diseases could be eliminated only by spiritual and mental effort. He described thirty-eight states of diseased soul and mind, and offered a remedy for each. Bach placed the main emphasis of cure on self-realization and spiritual progress.

About the flower essences, he stated that the action "is to raise our vibrations and to open up our channels for the reception of Spiritual Self."[11] His two main methods of preparation of his remedies were exposure to the sun and boiling. Although he called these methods "potentization," they obviously differ significantly from homeopathy.

According to many witnesses, Bach was an amazing healer. Always frail, he died in his sleep at age fifty. Bach remedies remain very popular. There's plenty of anecdotal evidence of their efficacy. But one thing is clear: they aren't homeopathy.

Anthroposophical Medicine

Austrian philosopher-scientist Rudolf Steiner founded a spiritual movement called anthroposophy, which incorporates a medical approach. He viewed humans as a system of four interconnected parts. He suggested that the physical body is related to minerals; the life force, called the "etheric body" by him, is related to plants; and the "astral body," represented by the emotions and the soul, is related to animals. According to Steiner, the human system also possesses a fourth important component: the "ego."

Anthroposophical medical treatment is highly individualized and only sometimes utilizes homeopathically prepared remedies. In addition, medications are prescribed according to principles different from those of classical homeopathy.

Homotoxicology

German physician Hans Heinrich Reckeweg formulated homotoxicology in 1952, presenting it as an attempt to create a "missing link" between homeopathy and allopathic medicine. In homotoxicology, diluted and potentized preparations are administered according to both allopathic indications and theoretical principles set forward by Reckeweg. He suggested that illnesses are caused by direct toxic influences of various substances and "nonmaterial." By this he meant influences like electromagnetic fields and "psychic" energy. He called influences *homotoxins*.

Reckeweg further hypothesized that homotoxins interact with each other or are processed in the liver to neutralize them. He called homotoxins that aren't eliminated through this process *retoxins*. Combined with homotoxins, these can affect the cells and tissues of the human body, triggering a process called *homotoxicosis*.

The goal of Reckeweg's treatment is to eliminate homotoxins, and assist the cells and tissues in elimination of retoxins deposited in their membranes. To accomplish these purposes, homotoxicology uses various preparations, including homeopathic remedies; conventional medications that are homeopathically prepared; enzymes; nosodes; and so-called Suis-organ preparations (homeopathically prepared organs and tissues of healthy pigs). Medications are administered both orally and through injections. This type of treatment is most probably suppressive in its action.

Homotoxicology is an attempt to use potentized remedies allopathically. But it isn't homeopathy in any shape or form. It has gained popularity with integrative physicians and their patients, and it's been incorporated into the more complex field of biological medicine, which draws upon elements of holistic dentistry, chelation, Western medicine, Eastern medicine, and homeopathy. At present, there's no evidence of its efficacy or lack thereof. Please remain aware of the risks of combining medications.

Homotoxicologists use injectable homeopathic remedies. Although these are potentized preparations of various substances, they don't represent homeopathy. Are they effective? Possibly. But if they are, they aren't different from allopathic medications. I'm not necessarily saying that they aren't helpful. Injectables are not homeopathy, that's all.

Homeopathic Drainage

French physician Léon Vannier developed homeopathic drainage between 1911 and the 1950s. This revisionist method of homeopathy is more popular in Europe than the United States. It is based on a hypothesis, rather than on direct research data, which presumes that the main issue in the disease process is the accumulation of toxins in the body. Also it incorporates polypharmacy, which is highly undesirable. Homeopathic drainage employs many homeopathic remedies simultaneously.

Vannier insisted that the choice of the drainage remedy should be individualized. In his process, the patient receives a "fundamental" remedy, which is selected based on a concept that's analogous, but not identical to the concept of the simillimum. On top of that, a nosode is always prescribed as a "regulating remedy." Then there are one or two "drainage" remedies in low potency, as well as "lesional" remedies directed towards regional problems. As a result, a patient may be receiving two remedies in high dilutions (200C), two in medium (30C), and one or two in low dilutions (6C). Remedies are usually administered in monthly "cycles" in increasing dilutions. They may also be changed according to the changes of symptoms.

Vannier also invented so-called prenatal homeopathy, by which he meant something quite different than giving pregnant women health care. Basically he suggested that instead of waiting for a child to be born with systemic conditions, one could administer nosodes to a pregnant mother to protect her child from future illnesses. He insisted that DNA could be modified in this way, and hereditary disease prevented. Unfortunately, there is no data to support or detract from this hypothesis.

Electrodiagnostic Machines

Some practitioners use electrodiagnostic devices to select homeopathic remedies. Proponents claim that the cause of disease is an "energy imbalance" that can be detected. They say such devices can diagnose diseases, including allergies and food sensitivities; vitamin deficiencies; asthma; cardiac problems; and even cancer and AIDS. Although they employ remedies, they often prescribe more than one, and in various potencies. They also use the devices to test the patient's need for supplements and allopathic medications.

In the early days, there was no computer present in this diagnostic system. The early devices were called Voll machines, and the procedure itself was called electroacupuncture according to Voll (EAV) or electrodermal screening (EDS). German physician Reinhold Voll developed the first device in 1958 so he could combine Chinese acupuncture theory with galvanic skin differentials in his system.

The main part of any EAV system is a galvanometer that measures the electrical resistance of the patient's skin when touched by a probe. The device emits a very low voltage (frequently below 1 volt) direct electric current. A wire from the device is connected to a brass cylinder that's covered by moist gauze. The patient holds this in one hand. A second wire is connected from the device to a probe, which the operator touches to various acupuncture points on the patient's other hand or a foot. This completes a low-voltage circuit and the device registers the flow of current.

The device is said to indicate the condition of a particular meridian, or energy channel, and its corresponding organs. This information is relayed to a gauge that provides a numerical readout on a scale of 0 to 100. Readings below 45 suggest organ stagnation and degeneration. Readings from 45 to 55 are considered normal and balanced. Readings above 55 indicate inflammation of the organ associated with the meridian being tested. The circuit includes a honeycomb cache in which glass ampules holding various preparations can be placed to "correct" for supposed deficiencies. The operator then observes changes on the dial and knows what remedy is indicated.

The original technique required examination of up to 850 acupuncture points. Then one of the Voll's students, Helmut Schimmel simplified the diagnostic system, made small modifications to the equipment, and created a new model, known as a Vegatest. There are many such devices on the market currently. All of them utilize computers. Nowadays, this technique is called bioelectric functions diagnosis (BFD), bioresonance therapy (BRT), or bioenergy regulatory technique (BER).

A complete examination for asthma or allergies may involve testing up to sixty acupuncture points, and involves miraculous readings for viral, bacterial, and chemical toxins. Then the computer suggests a list of potentially effective substances for treatment, including single and combination homeopathic remedies, nosodes, allergens, herbs, vitamins, minerals, and other items. These substances are then tested individually to determine which ones would allow the patient's body to return to a state of energetic harmony. Obviously, the ultimate prescription contains numerous components, including various homeopathic preparations.

The equipment is expensive. The evaluation is impressive and projects a flavor of "real" science and technology with multicolor schematic readouts on a computer screen. But this method is not homeopathy. Furthermore, its efficacy hasn't been adequately tested in controlled studies, and the ultimate treatment involves polypharmacy.

CHAPTER FIVE

Your Visit to the Homeopath

"'I'm one of the Sole Sanhedrims and Ostensible Hooplas of the Inner Pulpit,' says I. 'The lame talk and the blind rubber whenever I make a pass at 'em. I am a medium, a coloratura hypnotist and a spirituous control. It was only through me at the recent séances at Ann Arbor that the late president of the Vinegar Bitters Company could revisit the earth to communicate with his sister Jane.'"
—O. HENRY, *JEFF PETERS AS A PERSONAL MAGNET*

O. Henry's description perfectly fits the profile of a professional homeopath held in the minds of the majority of people who don't know much or anything about the field. Of course, that's not your understanding now, provided you've read the previous chapters. Even so, you may be surprised at what happens during a typical homeopathic evaluation, as well as by the types of questions a homeopath asks and, more importantly, doesn't ask. Many people have heard that homeopathy solves chronic health issues, and possibly they even know someone who was cured by a homeopath. Nonetheless, the inner workings of the homeopathic kitchen, so to speak, remain a mystery to them. This chapter therefore will address the realities of professional homeopathic practice.

In my experience, a large proportion of those who come to see a homeopath for the first time in their lives don't really know what to expect from treatment: how long it lasts, how homeopaths arrive at a particular remedy, what type of information the homeopathic practitioner considers, or how homeopathy interacts with other methods of treatment (both conventional and nonconventional). Very importantly, they also don't know how to find a good homeopathic practitioner.

Let's talk about these issues one at a time.

What Homeopathy Can and Can't Do for You and Your Family

First things first. What can and can't homeopathy do? In a small box, the answer is simple and clear: Homeopathy helps cure illnesses that result from potentially reversible malfunctions of the mind or the body. By this definition, a serious condition like depression or chronic asthma, or even a peptic ulcer may be cured, because in such cases, there is no permanent damage to the structural components of the body. Of course, no form of treatment can help to grow a new set of teeth or a new limb.

It is easy to appreciate the difference between these two types of situations (reversible and nonreversible), but what about conditions like cancer or serious, chronic illnesses for which a person comes to the homeopathic visit while taking one or more conventional medications. Will homeopathy work?

The main issue in whether or not homeopathic treatment is going to be successful is not how advanced or severe an illness is, or what you are taking for it, but how clearly a practitioner is able to identify the correct matching remedy to prescribe for it.

Providers of all kinds of alternative medicine are acutely aware of the fact that people often come to them with the expectations of an outcome close to a miracle, and the providers feel that they should deliver nothing short of a miracle every time they treat a patient. Homeopaths feel this way because we do get to see miracles, for real—but not each and every time. We see the miracle of cure only when the selection of a remedy is 100 percent accurate: when the entire unique picture of symptoms characteristic to the remedy fits the entire picture of the illness in a particular individual, the patient. Quite often, achieving such a precision in prescribing is not a one-shot deal. It requires an effort, not only on the part of the homeopath, but also on the part of the patient. Several visits may be required and several months may pass as the correct remedy is approached.

Another important factor in success is how many resources the patient possesses that support recovery. I have met cancer patients who were full of energy and hopes of recovery, and I have met young, strong looking men who were falling apart and demanding immediate relief from a sore throat. Resources are mental, emotional, and physical, and it can be surprising to discover who has got the most.

Although it would be inaccurate to produce a blanket statement covering all possible cases of illness, the rule of thumb is that there is going to be success in most cases where the physiological root is reversible. When there is no or little functional capacity left, such as in cases of hypothyroidism or insulin-dependent diabetes, we are really only talking about the possibility of decreasing the amount of conventional medications someone needs or palliation of their symptoms.

The Importance of Addressing Your Apparent Diseases

Since the days of Hahnemann, homeopaths have clearly distinguished what is called the *apparent disease* from other types of symptoms. This expression refers to the situation when the cause of an illness is clear and its removal will lead to a complete cure.

If I was working in an emergency room, and someone walked in with a knife sticking out of his back and told me: "Doc, I need you to cure me, but under no circumstances are you allowed to remove the knife," I wouldn't be able to help.

Yes, modern painkillers could remove the man's pain, but he would ultimately bleed to death or develop an infection that would kill him. To save him, it would be imperative for me to remove the knife, suture the wound, and make sure there was no damage done to his internal organs. Only after that could I promise him a cure.

I'll never forget the case of a middle-aged woman sent to me by referral from another homeopath. She had no appetite and was rapidly losing weight, had become weak and then developed severe digestive problems in combination with significant swelling in her legs. She waited a long time even to see a homeopath because she did not trust doctors. Based on many of the symptoms she presented, this homeopath, who also happens to be a family physician, strongly suspected the possibility of cancer and suggested the woman undergo a thorough medical workup. The patient refused even a regular physical exam. She stated that she did not trust "all these corrupt physicians."

In this case, the homeopath tried a few well-chosen homeopathic remedies without any effect. The patient was getting worse. Then the homeopath referred her to me. In a phone conversation we agreed that, based on all the symptoms she was exhibiting so far, a thorough medical workup was important. Fortunately, at the time I was working at Beth Israel, a medical center with good nurses. I spent literally an hour talking to the woman about the necessity of having a physical exam and doing many other studies. She finally agreed to be examined by a nurse. After collecting history and conducting an exam, the nurse advised the woman to seriously consider a full medical work up as she also suspected cancer. The woman returned to the first homeopath and eventually had some studies done that showed that she had an advanced stage of cancer. All the tests she needed were done too late.

The lesson of this unfortunate and not so exceptional case is simple. Doing nothing in cases when you have obviously alarming symptoms is dangerous. It is silly to deny the advances of modern biomedical science and concentrate only on negative information. You need to know what is going on in your body.

Interestingly, the notion that an infection is an apparent disease, and that simply killing a "bug" will lead to a cure for an infection is most probably wrong. First of all, not everyone becomes ill even during the worst epidemics of the most terrible illnesses. Secondly, even the most powerful antibiotics won't cure sick patients in 100 percent of cases. There is very little that antibiotics can do to kill viruses. An infectious disease is always a combination of an intrusion (being infected by bacteria or a virus) and a reaction from the host (a human being or an animal). Homeopathy helps make the host stronger so that the immune system can eliminate the intruder.

In my opinion, regular dental cleanings and checkups, and regular physicals, and pediatric or gynecological exams are a must. Knowing what's going on always puts you ahead of the game. Regardless of the diagnosis, you will always be in charge of making a decision what treatment to use. But you ought to be able to make an *informed* decision.

What Can You Expect During Treatment

I remember my first patient at the Continuum Center for Health and Healing at Beth Israel Hospital in New York very well. A Brazilian, she came to me with many serious chronic health issues, including probable infertility, PMS, and emotional problems. We spent two hours talking about her troubles, which, by the way, is a perfectly normal length of time for an initial homeopathic evaluation. At the end of the appointment, I started explaining the course of treatment. She interrupted: "Doctor, I grew up with homeopathy. I know that you'll give me only one dose of a highly diluted remedy and make me wait for a month or two before reassessing me."

I was pleasantly surprised. This type of a conversation had certainly not been the case with numerous patients I saw before in my practice in New York City. Most New Yorkers want results *now*, or, preferably, *yesterday*. Not that immediate results ever happen in real life with any type of treatment. But this is the attitude. Also people tend to feel that if something is good for you it must be taken every day, like a vitamin.

My Brazilian patient came back for her follow up visit a month later and reported that her mood was better, her premenstrual syndrome was 20 to 30 percent better, and her energy level had improved. Then she said: "From what I remember about homeopathy, I'm doing pretty well. There is slight, but definite progress."

I was totally blown away by her statement. She truly understood that the healing process, triggered by the homeopathic remedy, was going to proceed at the pace dictated by nature, not by either of our wishes.

This particular woman went on to improve significantly and, in the course of a year, gave birth to her first baby. Her husband, who became a believer in homeopathy after he saw his wife's improvement, came to see me for himself, and was cured of chronic migraine headaches. I lost track of their family a few years later.

A reality of homeopathic practice is that people get better and then disappear, which is appropriate if they're cured. Unfortunately, many patients who *don't* get better right away disappear, too. This is a big mistake!

What Information Is Important?

What can homeopaths do with all the different kinds of information that various other health care providers have offered you? Our approach to any kind of information should be pragmatic. If it helps to find the remedy, we need it. If it can't help us find the remedy, we should disregard it. Spending time talking about nonessential information actually decreases a homeopath's chance to find an appropriate remedy. After all, at least in my practice, the interview can last only for a limited amount of time (although long by conventional standards). So, what types of data are and what types of data are not important?

In my practice, I frequently hear a long list of information that an acupuncturist or ayurvedic doctor told my new patient. Unfortunately, other forms of medicine have little or no information that can be utilized by a homeopath, as our databases are not parallel. I cannot translate a report about weakness of chi in the liver meridian into finding an apt remedy. Telling me about an excess of any of the three doshas will also do us no good. I respect Chinese medicine and ayurveda. I have seen people get good results from them. But there are no practical bridges between them and homeopathy. Homeopathy developed in western culture and is based on a different theoretical foundation.

What about conventional medical information? Can a homeopath utilize data derived from modern biomedical examination? Yes, with the qualifier: to a certain extent. Here's why.

Both systems—homeopathy and allopathy, or conventional medicine—officially recognize that illness affects the entire human being, but only homeopathy puts this idea into practice. As we all know, specialization is the middle name of modern medicine. Psychologists and psychiatrists stand apart from the other disjointed medical specialists who either totally ignore their patients' emotional states or "throw" an antidepressant at them. A homeopath is acutely aware of the utmost importance of the emotional state created by illness. While conventional medicine emphasizes having a detailed understanding of local changes in different organs and systems of our body, such as the brain and nervous system, homeopathy pays more attention to the systemic reaction of the entire human being to the illness, such as migraine headaches.

A patient who suffers from migraine headaches will have to undergo a series of imaging studies of the brain, detailed neurological evaluations, and numerous blood tests. If all of these tests come back negative, a conventional medical doctor will offer the patient a medication based on the rate of success he or she has had in using it for treatment of uncomplicated migraines in the past.

A homeopath will be similarly interested to learn that this patient's headache is not caused by a tumor, a brain hemorrhage, or any other apparent cause, but then will want to collect additional data to determine how different this particular individual with headaches is from everyone else with the same diagnosis. The homeopath will ask questions about which side the headache is, the timing and the triggers of the headache, and the emotional characteristics of the person. Even food desires and aversions will be examined to establish a unique picture of the illness in this particular individual. Those symptoms will then be matched with a remedy. Homoeopathy has a high degree of precision as provings have been done on over 2500 homeopathic remedies.

After reading all that, hopefully it is clear that while lab work and the results of an MRI are important for developing a clear idea of what damage, if any, has been done on a physical level, they still are just small pieces of the health puzzle. A much larger and most important section of the puzzle for a homeopath is the information about the *reaction* of the whole human being to the illness or damage.

What does this mean for your visit? A homeopath will appreciate any test results that you bring to the office, but please do not spend too much time talking about them, and certainly spend even less time discussing your conventional medications. Again, a homeopath needs to know about drugs you're taking, but the logic of a conventional physician is not so important to us. Not because it is wrong, but because it is different and cannot become a part of the database. By *database*, I mean the collection of bits of information that will ultimately lead to the selection of a remedy.

Be prepared to describe your food preferences, the position in which you like to sleep, your fears, your dreams, and activities you like to do for fun. A homeopath will spend a lot of time trying to understand what natural things make your symptoms better or worse, such as the time of the day, positions, and the temperature. All these bits of information make you different from everyone else experiencing the same complaint.

On any given day, I may see a few patients with migraine headaches and prescribe different remedies for each one of them because of the fact that what triggers their headaches, the precise location of their pain, the things that make them feel better or worse, and the type of personality they each have are different.

On the other hand, I may wind up giving the same remedy to a few people with different diseases. For example, Nancy, a beautiful, shy five-year-old with severe asthma told me her asthma feels worse inside of the house and always gets better outdoors. Each time she has an asthma attack, she has to sit propped-up in bed, becomes tearful, and wants her mommy to hold her and say nice things to her. Her asthma is worse at night. Nancy cries easily, and often asks her parents: "Do you love me?" She sleeps on her back and always sticks her feet out from under the covers. She cannot stay in the sun because she gets too hot and may even faint. She also loves creamy things. Her mother told me that Nancy can eat butter with a spoon. There were many other characteristics I learned in our first visit, and all pointed clearly to a homeopathic remedy named *Pulsatilla nigricans* that cured Nancy's asthma.

A while ago I also saw Jack, a fifty-year-old biker sporting numerous tattoos and a beard. Jack is a big guy. He pumps iron. He likes to wear leather and chains, and talks in a deep voice. He visited a urologist, complaining of frequent urination. The urologist diagnosed him with prostatitis (an inflammation of the prostate) and prescribed antibiotics. However, a few courses of antibiotics brought about only temporary relief.

Interestingly, this big guy came to see me in the company of his wife of thirty years. During the interview I quickly discovered that this menacing-looking man is actually pretty tender, loves to spend time with his wife, and loves his three daughters. Every time he doesn't feel well, he needs his wife to hold him and tell him how much she loves him. He constantly feels warm and needs the air conditioning to blast all summer. Unfortunately, this creates problems for his wife who is exactly the opposite way. Jack sleeps on his back and always kicks the covers off. He cannot stay out in the sun because it gives him headaches. His frequent urination problem is worse at night. He also *loves* to eat butter and strawberries with a lot of cream.

Like little Nancy, I gave Jack *Pulsatilla nigricans* with excellent results.

Interestingly, other people who love butter, or are warm-blooded, or cry easily, but otherwise have totally different characteristics would need different remedies. The same is true for their illnesses. Not everyone with asthma needs *Pulsatilla nigricans,* and men with prostate problems require all different kinds of remedies. The unique combination of all the symptoms someone shows me is the key to finding the remedy—not just one thing.

What Tools Do Homeopaths Use?

You will notice that most contemporary homeopaths use computers. How does this help us find a remedy? Professional homeopathic software contains two main types of books. *Materia Medica*, the Latin title for a book on pharmacology, as discussed in Chapter 2, contains detailed information about each remedy. Another type of book is a repertory. There are many different ones. Each is an index of all the possible symptoms that have been registered by homeopaths, either in provings or from being cured, during use of a particular remedy.

Both types of books compile a massive database that, before the computer age, had to be studied "by hand." The computer allows us to handle our searches more efficiently, as modern programs offer searchable libraries equivalent to hundreds of thick books. What the computer cannot do, however, is find a remedy for you. A good British edition that I own of the main repertory by American homeopath James Tyler Kent has lost its front cover from my extensive use. Then I bought the currently popular repertory *Synthesis,* which now also shows clear indications of wear. Identifying and cross-referencing noteworthy symptoms, and choosing remedies, remain important skills that each homeopath has to gain from many years of continuous study and clinical experience.

Don't be fooled by various web sites on the internet that promise an easy way to find the remedy you need. Also don't be fooled by methods whereby a computer is directly "hooked" to a patient and allegedly measures some kind of a biological field or "diagnoses" Chinese meridians and finds the remedy based on that. As yet, no reliable correlation has been made between Chinese medicine and homeopathy. Another consideration is that these types of software always seem to come up with a huge list of different supplements, herbs, and various homeopathic preparations that a single person should take. Well, here we go again! That's prescribing multiple medications with unknown interactions with both our body and each other.

If it still sounds like a good idea, go for it! Clearly, I have my doubts.

Finding a Good Homeopath

The time has come to answer the "million-dollar question": How does someone like you find a good homeopath? My answer is not complicated. Basically, you only have two good choices. The first and best option is to go to a homeopath recommended by a friend who has had a good experience with this particular practitioner. Seek satisfied customers. The second option is to consult one of the field's professional organizations.

Let's discuss these associations and schools, and their degrees and accreditations.

Different countries have unique regulations about the practice of homeopathy. In some countries, like France, Italy, Russia, India, and a few nations in South America, only highly trained medical professionals can practice homeopathy. In France, Italy, and Russia: only physicians. India has over 200,000 homeopathic doctors, and my understanding is that there are two levels of training and degrees, one equal to an M.D. and the other on a par with a physician's assistant (P.A.).

England and Germany have specialized education and licensing for homeopaths: One is permitted to be a physician and also practice homeopathy. Many industrialized countries, for example England, France, and Germany, have integrated homeopathy into their national health system. Personally, I am familiar with claim forms that German and French patients ask me to sign to receive full reimbursement for homeopathic services.

The situation in the United States is more complicated. At the time of this writing, only three states—Arizona, Connecticut, and Nevada—license homeopathic practitioners. In Connecticut, homeopaths have to be M.D.s and sit for a multiple-choice exam. For a passing score they are granted the title *homeopathic physician.* In Arizona and Nevada both M.D.s and M.D.-supervised non-M.D.s are permitted to practice homeopathy. Many states recognize naturopathic doctors (N.D.) as practicing medicine legally, and some of the N.D.s (but far from all of them!) practice homeopathy. Other states do not explicitly prohibit homeopathy, yet they do not provide a specific certification process.

A recent movement for the freedom of choice in medical treatment has created legislative measures in some states that allow anyone to practice homeopathy. Homeopathic training is provided either by some naturopathic schools as a part of a larger comprehensive curriculum or by independent privately run part-time homeopathic schools. These schools accept students from any background, including M.D.s, N.D.s, nurse practitioners, chiropractors, acupuncturists, and laypeople.

Medical doctors practicing homeopathy belong to a professional organization known as the American Institute of Homeopathy (AIH), which in 1844 was the first professional medical organization established in the U.S. Naturopathic doctors likewise have their own organization, the Homeopathic Academy of Naturopathic Physicians (HANP), which was established in 1982. An organization called the North American Society of Homeopaths (NASH) was founded in 1990 with a membership that's a mixture of non-licensed (majority) and licensed practitioners. Members of this organization call themselves professional homeopaths, but, as you learned already, their training actually does not differ from members of other organizations.

There are three major homeopathic boards in the United States. The American Board of Homeotherapeutics (ABHt) was established by the AIH in 1959. There is also a board of HANP established in the 1980s. A Council of Homeopathic Certification (CHC) was created in 1991 to establish a "certification of competency in homeopathy." As of today, none of these certifications provides a license to practice homeopathy. Although there is an ongoing effort to provide a unified certification process, at the moment the ABHT continues to use its own format. All the certification organizations offer a four-part process that includes the review of credentials and training, review of records of about ten cured cases, a written multiple choice, and an oral exam. The process is entirely voluntary, expensive, and laborious. I went through the ABHt certification process myself and I have to report that it was the most difficult exam I ever took in my life.

The current board of directors of a large organization called the National Center for Homeopathy (NCH) has been working in accord with all the other homeopathic organizations in the United States to provide a climate conducive to collaboration and, ultimately, to better standards of homeopathic care. There is also an ongoing effort to create a full-time fully accredited homeopathic medical school in the State of Arizona.

The Council on Homeopathic Education (CHE) was established in 1982 as an independent agency to assess homeopathic training in the United States and Canada. It has become significantly more active in recent years. Homeopaths have great hopes that the Council's relentless activity will result in a significant improvement in the quality of homeopathic education. The number of schools accredited by CHE is rapidly growing.

In my opinion, claims by the members of one organization or another that their level of proficiency in homeopathy is higher than members of other organizations are subjective. At the end of the day, you, the consumer, are left with the freedom to choose anyone whom you believe suits your particular situation. I don't feel qualified to endorse or denounce any type of practitioners. The choice ultimately remains yours.

Each of the above organizations has websites that offer detailed information on their guiding principles and individual practitioners.

As you read on in *Easy Homeopathy,* you'll be given the opportunity to choose from among seven main remedies and dozens of secondary remedies when you're confronting different emerging and everyday health challenges. If ever you feel confused when making your decision about what remedy to apply, it is perfectly OK—and perhaps even advisable—to seek the counsel of a trained homeopath. I think you'll find, however, that the information in this book is remarkably useable.

In due course, you'll become familiar with these seven remedies and understand their role in your daily life.

CHAPTER SIX

Instructions for Using Homeopathic Remedies

When all else fails, read the instructions.

This chapter is a set of instructions on how to use remedies correctly.

When to Administer Your Homeopathic Remedy

It is essential to take your homeopathic remedy at least twenty minutes apart from strongly flavored items such as food, beverages (excluding water), smoking, toothpaste, and other medications.

Allow one to two minutes between each homeopathic remedy to optimize its effects.

The reasoning behind these couple of administration guidelines is that the efficacy of homeopathic remedies is believed to be enhanced through absorption in the mouth lining, and strong flavors may interfere with this absorption.

Taking Your Homeopathic Remedy

Most commonly homeopathic remedies come in the form of a pill. These come packaged either in a glass vial or a plastic tube that has a special cap you twist to dispense the remedy. Minimize contact with your hands, as the pills are coated with the homeopathic remedy.

For pills that come in glass bottles, tip them into the bottle cap or onto a clean spoon and then transfer them to your mouth. Hold in the mouth for at least ten seconds before sucking or chewing. Do not swallow with water.

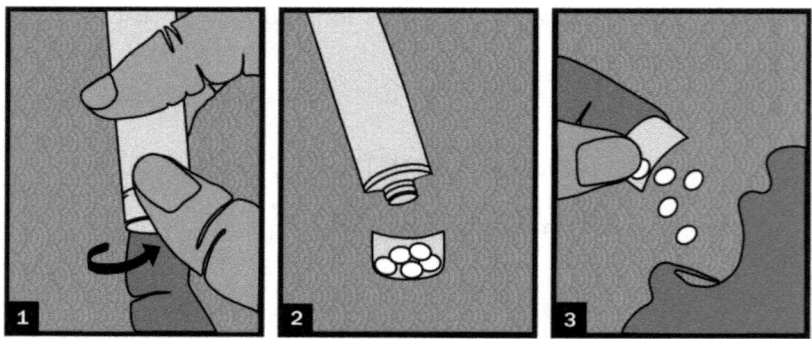

In using homeopathic tubes:
1. Turn the tube upside down so that the clear cap is at the bottom.
2. Twist the clear cap until the required number of pills drop into it.
3. Tip the pills from the cap into your mouth.
4. Replace the cap.

How to Give Remedies to Babies and Young Children

For babies and young children:
- Crush the pills or tablets between two clean spoons and then place the resulting powder directly onto the child's tongue.
- You can also dilute pills in a small amount of water before giving them to your baby to swallow.

Storage of Remedies

Store remedies in a cool, dry place away from direct sunlight and strong-smelling substances such as camphor, menthol, soaps, eucalyptus, and perfumes. Keep remedies away from electronic gadgets, mobile phones, and other radiation-emitting equipment if possible. Always store medicines out of the sight and reach of children.

Duration of Remedy Use

The duration of taking a remedy varies for each individual—and for each condition that's being treated. Aim for a steady improvement in symptoms. If symptoms disappear completely, stop taking your homeopathic remedy. Or follow your doctor's instructions.

Possible Reactions to Your Remedy

Homeopathy is a safe and gentle healing method, working differently than conventional medicines. Occasionally, homeopathic treatment may cause a flare-up, known as an *aggravation,* which is typically a positive sign. If you experience an aggravation, pause the medicine until the flareup settles. If it persists, contact your homeopathic pharmacy.

PART TWO

SUPER REMEDIES

CHAPTER SEVEN

Stramonium Your Savior

"PTSD. It's not the person refusing to let go if the past, but the past refusing to let go of the person."
—UNKNOWN AUTHOR

ATTENTION! If you were a victim of severe abuse, rape, or assault or you were traumatized by participating in military actions and/or witnessing horrific events, reading this chapter might trigger a strong emotional response. I suggest you allow someone you trust, who has no such history, to read the chapter and tell you the essence of what they've read. It would be ideal if such a person were your therapist. The remedy described in this chapter is known to help in many cases of severe PTSD, but as is the case with all other homeopathic remedies, the individual who needs this remedy is very likely to be hypersensitive to even hearing a description of the symptoms it treats.

You may have noticed that the other super remedies in this book are listed in alphabetic order. Letter S, with which this remedy's name begins, is the nineteenth letter in the English alphabet, yet I am covering this remedy first. It is *that* important, and much needed these days. Illustrated alphabets for children often put a picture of a sunflower, a star, or a snake next to a giant S to help children remember the letter. But I suggest we use a different mnemonic for this remedy: the word *suffering.*

Just to make it crystal clear from the beginning, from now on you may want to think about *Stramonium* as the main remedy for severe, *chronic* post-traumatic stress disorder (PTSD) and about *Aconitum napellus* (described in the next chapter) as the main remedy for *acute* PTSD. I find this distinction so meaningful that I've decided to expand the explanation. For example, imagine you are at a beautiful resort by the ocean and a horrible storm with a horrible flood is breaking out right in front of you. You feel scared shitless, like it is the end of the world and you need to run for your life. In homeopathy, THAT is what we would call an *Aconitum* STATE and the remedy you'll need to cure these symptoms should they stay with you after you escape would be *Aconitum.*

On the other hand, if you witnessed the very same event and now some time has elapsed and you've developed severe chronic flashbacks, severe nightmares, fear of the dark, and a sense of hypervigilance (a feeling of being on high alert, as if there is an imminent danger), your thoughts should lean more toward *Stramonium.*

Hundreds of my patients developed a *Stramonium* state after going through the experience of September 11, 2001. (We simply call it 9/11 in the United States. Nine-eleven.) I presented some of these cured cases at the LIGA Medicorum conference in Berlin in 2003.

It is likely that a large number of people who were initially caught up in the 9/11 disaster felt extremely scared, like they were going to **die right now,** and were compelled to run away, and that they were shaky and fearful while telling their stories to friends and relatives afterward— still feeling like they were in imminent danger, going to die, and needed to move, or even to run away. But I wasn't there to give them a dose of

Aconitum, nor did they know about it. So, it is probably too late for them to take *Aconitum.*

What they are more likely to need today, if they are still feeling triggered or haunted by a traumatic event from the past, is *Stramonium.*

Now you know the difference between the timing of the two remedies. And you are about to learn about *Stramonium,* a remedy needed for a much deeper, much darker state that might feel like hell.

Before I get further into it, I need to make another important point about this chapter on Stramonium. In homeopathy there is no such thing as "a remedy for PTSD" or "a remedy for asthma." Remedies align with states not with diseases. Yes, *Stramonium* is frequently required and appropriate for the treatment of PTSD with homeopathy, but it will be effective *only* if the person who has been diagnosed with PTSD has characteristics and symptoms known to be associated with a *Stramonium* state. There are going to be a lot of these people. But there are also going to be a lot of other people who need to take a dose of something else. So, if you do not see a clear picture that calls for *Stramonium,* don't use it. Of course, it is always better to consult with a professional homeopath.

As any other homeopathic remedy, *Stramonium* can be helpful in addressing a large number and variety of conditions—as along as the core symptoms a person is experiencing correspond to the core characteristics of the *Stramonium* state. As long as the essence of the condition is the same. For example, *Stramonium* was frequently used in olden times for the treatment of severe fever in children that was accompanied with elements of violence. (Please do not jump ahead, however, and try *Stramonium* for fevers before you read the chapters on *Aconitum* and *Belladonna.*)

Stramonium is also frequently used by contemporary homeopaths who treat autistic children (when they present with severe nightmares, elements of violence, and various other symptoms that are characteristic for the *Stramonium* state).

Very importantly, this chapter is dedicated to using *Stramonium* to help people with PTSD. I decided to concentrate on how to treat the horrible PTSD epidemic that our world is experiencing at present.

Whereas every other chapter contains flowcharts helping us understand alternative homeopathic remedies for various acute conditions, this chapter is dedicated exclusively to helping people with chronic PTSD. No flow charts, just a comparison with only one other remedy *Aconitum*, which has its own chapter fully dedicated to presenting various options for various acute conditions.

I know I said it just a few lines above, but the point is so critically important that I feel I must repeat it. If you (or someone you are trying to help) feel like your life is in imminent danger, if you feel a strong impulse to move or run away, or if your face is showing an expression of severe fear, then think *Aconitum*.

If you (or someone you are trying to help) went through a life-threatening experience and/or witnessed a horrible event and now has severe nightmares, flashbacks, gets easily angered, and has many fears, then consider taking *Stramonium*.

The Origins of *Stramonium*

Stramonium (*Datura stramonium*, or simply datura), also known as devil's trumpets, hell's bells, thorn apple, and jimsonweed, is a delicate annual herb or herbaceous perennial belonging to the nightshade family of plants (*Solanaceae*). For our discussion, such relatively rare names of this plant as devil's horn and hell's bells are important to remember, as they describe the main theme of the emotional state that requires this remedy. But the most commonly used names for the plant in the English-speaking world are thorn apple and jimsonweed.

Characterized by a green to purplish stem emitting an unpleasant odor, this plant features alternate, simple, coarsely toothed leaves. Its solitary flowers are large and tubular, with five shallow lobes at the top, appearing in white or lavender hues. Notably, these fragrant flowers open at night, attracting nocturnal moths.

This plant thrives in disturbed areas, along roadsides, old fields, pastures, and waste places, often infiltrating gardens as an unwelcome weed.

While a homeopathic preparation of *Stramonium* is harmless and can cure many cases of severe illness, being poisoned with the plant or its juices produces unpleasant, potentially dangerous symptoms.

Consumption of raw leaves and seeds can result in severe poisoning, manifesting in symptoms such as hot, dry, and flushed skin, hallucinations, pupil dilation, headaches, delirium, a rapid and weak pulse, convulsions, and, in extreme cases, coma. It is crucial to exercise caution and awareness regarding the presence of Jimsonweed in various environments, recognizing its potential hazards and taking appropriate measures to prevent accidental ingestion.

The datura flower holds immense significance among Hindus due to its legendary association with a powerful deity. According to ancient scriptures and beliefs, this flower grew from Lord Shiva's chest after he drank poison during a battle between the devas (gods) and the asuras (demons). This poison, which is known as *halahal* or *kalakuta,* emerged during the churning of the ocean (the *samudra manthan),* which was a great threat to the three worlds of heaven, earth, and hell. To save all living beings, Lord Shiva drank the poison, which turned his neck blue, giving him the nickname Neelakanth (the "blue-necked one").

That the datura plant is alternately known as devil's trumpets, devil's weed, and hell's bells is appropriate for the homeopathic remedy made from it because symptoms that can be treated by *Stramonium* usually begin after all hell breaks loose. A large number of people with severe PTSD benefit from taking this remedy. And I dare to say that since COVID, *horror* and *disaster* are the best single word definitions of our time. Figuratively speaking, we have all been hearing the bells of hell! Sometimes it looks like we are cosplaying the movie *Joker* that came out in 2019 right before COVID started. I remember saying to myself while watching that movie, "I hope this sick fantasy won't become our reality!"

Nope. It has been playing out in real life in front of us. *Stramonium* has become one of the most important homeopathic remedies of our times. And what a scary, horrible time this is! Between the ongoing and increased levels of violence and political and economic turmoil in almost every country in the world, including major wars in Israel and the Ukraine, millions of people are simultaneously suffering from post-trauma. Conventional medicine and psychology do offer some solutions for the symptoms, but these solutions are far from ideal, and they take a long time to start relieving the severe inner suffering that is characteristic of this condition. While homeopathic *Stramonium* is not a magic wand at all, in my extensive experience in treating severe PTSD, it can provide fast, effective relief of its major and most disturbing symptoms.

In homeopathy, *Stramonium* is well known for being helpful to children, who suffer from such severe emotional problems as night terrors and violent behavior. Of course, as is the case for most homeopathic remedies, one remedy is not suitable for all individual cases, so I am going to provide some alternatives. I would like to emphasize that while in some cases a few doses of *Stramonium* can be all that a person needs to get over the most disturbing aspects of their PTSD presentation, seeking professional help from both a homeopath and a psychologist is highly recommended. In many severe cases, the involvement of a professional psychiatrist could also be necessary. Be assured, however, that healing is possible.

Symptoms Characteristic of the *Stramonium* State

Any condition that begins with the following unique combination of circumstances followed by symptoms listed below can be helped with *Stramonium*.

For adults:

- Exposure to a life-threatening event, severe violence.
- Deep-seated fear that is easily triggered by even the slightest of stresses.
- Fear of the dark, water, or dogs.
- Flashbacks of traumatic events.
- Severe nightmares.
- Expressions of agression ranging from being easily irritated to becoming verbally and physically violent at the least possible provocation (the violence could even be provoked by someone disagreeing with an opinion).
- Hypervigilance.

While an experienced homeopath might be able to prescribe *Stramonium* for complicated, not so obvious cases, it has been my experience that an overwhelming majority of people who benefited from *Stramonium* presented with a very clear set of symptoms and circumstances that triggered their condition.

In my opinion, an excellent illustration of the state of *Stramonium* is the story of one of my patients, a man whom I will call Richard though this is not his real name.

Before I start describing real cases of my patients, I would like to tell you something very important. Probably what I'm about to say is one of the most important messages I'd like you to take away from reading this book. THERE IS NO ONE-PILL-CURE-IT-ALL solution for complex, deeply internalized problems. Neither emotional ones, nor physical ones. An effective, wisely chosen remedy or conventional medication may create a solid foundation for the healing process to begin. But there are many other important steps that need to be taken in order to get to the high point of cure.

In my opinion, this remedy should be on the World Health Organization's Essential Medicines List because it is the most frequently used and highly effective homeopathic remedy for PTSD, especially following nightmares and violence.

As promised I am going to tell you about Richard, one of my first post-9/11 patients. Richard had the misfortune of being present for both the 1993 and the 2001 World Trade Center (WTC) terrorist attacks. On the morning of September 11, 2001, Richard was in a subway station under the WTC when the first airplane hit the North Tower at 8:46 AM. Evacuated with everyone else, he realized that he had left his attaché case at the subway station. So, he went back, crawled into the station in the dark, retrieved the case, and went to his office in a building right across from the Twin Towers. There, he stayed glued to the window and watched the bodies of people jumping out of a building to escape the fire flying through the air until both towers collapsed an hour and a half later. The images of these people had stayed with him day and night ever since.

When we met in 2002, he told me that he had become progressively more withdrawn. He was morbidly afraid of the dark, had terrible nightmares and flashbacks. Usually a mild-mannered man, he also had become extremely argumentative. At one point two young men attempted to mug him at gunpoint in a parking lot near his home. He disarmed them and actually bit them viciously until the police came. Even then, he had to be pulled away from the criminals.

Richard was unable to sleep at all because of constant nightmares. He felt very guilty that he was still alive while his colleagues and friends from the Trade Center were dead. He lost his ability to concentrate. A prominent computer analyst, he was being paid a high salary, but was unable to perform his job.

Two weeks after taking a single dose of *Stramonium* 200C, Richard came to my office for a follow-up visit and reported having no nightmares for the previous five days.

Four weeks later, he came to see me again and told me that in the course of the six weeks since the first dose of the remedy he'd only had two nightmares, his mood was much better, and he felt significantly less irritable.

As you probably figured now, at the initial evaluation I felt strongly that Richard was displaying all the symptoms of post-traumatic stress disorder. PTSD is a psychiatric disorder that can occur following the experience of witnessing life-threatening events, such as military combat, natural disasters, terrorist incidents, serious accidents, or violent personal assaults, like rape. People who suffer from PTSD often relive the experience through nightmares and flashbacks, have difficulty sleeping, and feel detached or estranged; and these symptoms can be severe enough and last long enough to significantly impair the person's daily life.

A PTSD mnemonic is:
- Event/experience is threatening to life or physical integrity of self or others),
- Reexperiencing the event (flashbacks, nightmares, daydreams),
- Arousal (anxiety, startle, hypervigilance, irritability),
- Avoidance (of things, places, people, and images reminiscent of the event), and,
- Duration of one month-plus.

Here is the story of another patient I was able to help with *Stramonium*. During an intake evaluation conducted by me at my psychiatric office, an older gentleman whom we are going to call Elliot complained of feeling very anxious and irritable. This seemingly mild-mannered, respectful gentleman related to me that his angry outbursts had been creating issues in his relationships with his wife, children, grandchildren, friends, and members of the temple to which he belonged. Elliot had heard that some antianxiety and antidepressant medications could be helpful. One of his wife's girlfriends also recommended that he ask me about Xanax.

As a part of my routine psychiatric evaluation, I took a history. I asked Elliot what kind of work he was doing. He responded: "I used to be a photographer, but I can't work anymore." Explaining the reason for this, he continued, "A few years ago, a man walked into my photography shop with an axe and told me and my partner to give him all the money we had in our cash register. After we gave him the cash, he broke the glass display counter and demanded we hand him our expensive cameras.

"I served in the military and know how to fight, so instead of complying, I told him to go away. He attacked me with with his axe. I fought back. My partner was able to call 911 as this was happening. By the time police came and arrested him, the robber managed to wound my shoulder badly. They had to perform surgery at the hospital.

"I have not been myself ever since. Horrible nightmares do not let me sleep, and I always feel that someone will attack me. Even the smallest contradiction in conversation drives me mad."

What would you, my inexperienced student, reckon I told Elliot to do? Did you say I advised him to take *Stramonium*?

Well, my situation was not simple. At the time of Elliot's evaluation, I was wearing the hat of a conventional psychiatrist. In front of me I had a patient who came for psychiatric medication and knew nothing about homeopathy. Giving him a lecture on homeopathy at that moment was not a very good idea.

This is what I did instead. First, I explained why I thought Elliot had been suffering from severe PTSD. Then I explained what pharmaceutical medications I could prescribe for his severe anxiety, insomnia, and nightmares. Elliot asked a few clarifying questions and we developed a plan. Then I wrote him a few prescriptions.

Elliot seemed very pleased with this outcome.

We had spent an hour-plus together, and it was evident that he liked me and felt comfortable with me. Given this, I also felt comfortable enough to mention that there was a natural remedy made out of a plant that might be able to help him with the issues that were troubling him, including the severe nightmares. He was interested to learn more.

I described *Stramonium* and suggested that he go home and buy a 30C tube of it on Amazon and try it for a few days. If it didn't work, then he could start taking the allopathic medications I'd just prescribed.

As you've probably guessed, a few doses of *Stramonium* changed the whole picture for Elliot. We continued seeing each other every few months to make sure he was OK. There were a few stressful situations in this period that triggered some nightmares and anxiety, but one or two doses of *Stramonium* took care of those.

Unfortunately, during the COVID pandemic Elliot lost a few family members and became extremely depressed. At that point, I supported his decision to take an antidepressant. But to this day, every time his nightmares come back, Elliot takes a few doses of *Stramonium*.

A Few Words of Wisdom

If you are in doubt, and don't know what remedy to choose, do not choose anything. While no big harm would be done by taking a wrong remedy, it might delay help you or your loved one needs right away. Please remember, this book is not about choosing homeopathy over nonhomeopathic treatment. It is about trying out a natural remedy during the window of opportunity you have when you are on your way to your doctor or the ER. Please do not hesitate to get the help you need!

Also, please understand that a person who went through a traumatic experience years ago can remain stuck in seemingly acute state of *Aconitum*. Even years later, they may on occasion feel extremely scared and agitated with a need to escape or run away.

On the other hand, a person who just went through an extremely traumatic experience can go immediately into the *Stramonium* state, becoming easily angered and developing severe nightmares, flashbacks, fear of the dark, fear of dogs, fear of water, and feeling an overall sense of horrible doom and gloom.

The next chapter of this book is dedicated to *Aconitum*, a remedy that was mentioned a few times in this chapter. That and all the chapters following it will contain flowcharts for assessing various acute conditions that offer you alternatives to the main remedy to which the chapter is dedicated.

I did not do any of that for *Stramonium*. The only other remedy mentioned here is *Aconitum*. I did it on purpose as I know from my vast experience that we all be much better off by just paying attention to people who clearly need *Stramonium*. There have been many and, unfortunately even more will come out way due to many horrible events that have been happening in the world.

There are some key differences between *Stramonium* and *Aconitum*. We use *Aconitum* similarly to the way an emergency services unit responds immediately to the scene of a crisis to treat the initial stages of the sort of **intense terror** and **restless anxiety**—to the degree of fearing imminent death—that often appear after experiencing or directly witnessing a horrific event, such as a terrible car crash, a murder, an act of terrorism, or another form of violent crime. By comparison, *Stramonium* becomes helpful usually at a later time, when, if left untreated, all the horror and the darkness has gone deeper. A person who needs *Stramonium* usually does not feel constant imminent threat to their life, does not need to move and run away. All the horror the person witnessed and/or went through goes very deep, causing severe night terrors and an overwhelming, ongoing feeling of darkness.

When *Not* to Self-Medicate with *Stramonium*

Best to try a different remedy if:
- A person is resistant to receiving any kind of help. I know it may sound silly to you on first reading this remark, but please stop for a moment and think about how many times you've offered

assistance to people and they rejected your help for various reasons. This kind of experience is especially true with homeopathy as many people have never heard of it or believe that it is fake medicine.

- The person is diagnosed with a serious chronic condition of any kind and is taking medication already.
- There is no history of severe emotional trauma such as was described at the beginning of the chapter. Although there have been thousands of cases cured with *Stramonium* when there was no apparent history of trauma (mostly in children), those cases require professional involvement and you should not interfere.
- You, or a person you intend to recommend Stramonium or any other homeopathic remedy to, are pregnant or breastfeeding. Although homeopathic remedies don't have side effects, when you are pregnant or breastfeeding the amount of time that you can safely spend trying to self-medicate with various remedies is significantly less, so please seek the advice of a health care professional immediately.

CHAPTER EIGHT

Aconitum

Your Homeopathic Emergency Services Unit

"Excessive fear is always powerless."
—AESCHYLUS

*A*conitum napellus (aconite, monkshood, wolf's bane) represents the first line of homeopathic defense against a set of serious symptoms. Hopefully, you and your family will never need it. But if you do, it's incredibly valuable.

We use *Aconitum* similarly to the way an emergency services unit responds immediately to the scene of a crisis. This remedy is used to treat the initial stages of a **head cold**, **flu**, or any other **acute illness** that's characterized by a sudden onset of symptoms, and accompanied by fear and restlessness. Children in the earliest stage of **croup**, for instance, may become extremely frightened and agitated as their throats narrow. It is also used to treat the sort of **intense terror** and **restless anxiety**—to the degree of fearing imminent death—that often appear after experiencing or directly witnessing a horrific event, such as a terrible car crash, a murder, an act of terrorism, or another form of violent crime.

The Origins of Aconite

Aconitum napellus is an impressive plant. Roughly four to five feet tall and decorated with a thick bunch of dark blue blossoms arranged in a spike, the plant usually grows in damp, shady spots in the mountains and flowers during the peak of summer. Since the shape of the flowers is reminiscent of a hood thrown over the head of a monk, the plant is commonly called monkshood.

In Sanskrit, an ancient tongue of Asia, the plant is called by the names *ativisha* and *visha*. Both words mean "poison." The word *aconite* is derived from the Ancient Greek word *akon*, meaning "dart," which refers to arrows poisoned with the juices of the plant. *Wolf's bane* refers to its early use as poison bait for wolves. In the Middle Ages, aconite was even believed to protect against werewolves. Long ago, in some cultures, women were known to use the plant's extracts to poison their unfaithful husbands.

While a homeopathic preparation of aconite is harmless and can cure many cases of severe illness, being poisoned with the plant or its juices produces terrible symptoms. As the root of the plant closely resembles horseradish, in the remote past accidental poisonings with the root were relatively common. The plant was also a popular source of poison for political intrigues. Even before conducting a proving, Samuel Hahnemann already knew many of the symptoms aconite would produce simply because they had been described in literature for many years.

John Henry Clarke, M.D., a renowned British homeopath, working at the turn of the twentieth century, once said, "Aconite is one of the deadliest and most readily acting poisons, yet, through Hahnemann's discoveries, it has been transformed into the best friend of the nursery."[1] He was referring to the remedy's success in treating croup.

For a poison to be truly effective, it has to produce symptoms quickly, and those symptoms have to be intense enough to lead to death. This is especially true for poisons used in hunting or combat situations. Certainly, plotting the murder of a rival, whether political or romantic, includes an expectation of tremendous suffering by the victim before he or she dies. Aconite poisoning fits this profile perfectly. Its symptoms come on **suddenly** and with **great intensity**. The victim experiences **tremendous anxiety**, **violent fear**, and **restlessness**. The **face feels very hot** and there is **tremendous thirst**. Victims of such symptoms die from respiratory and cardiac arrest.

The symptoms of poisoning lead us in identifying the symptoms characteristic to people who benefit from taking Aconitum as a remedy. As you can clearly see, all the reactions are fairly violent, intense, and sudden. The famous American homeopath James Tyler Kent described the picture of an Aconitum state in the following way: "All these . . . conditions are attended with great excitement of the circulation, violent action of the heart, a tremendous turmoil of the brain, a violent shock with intense fear."[2]

Symptoms Characteristic of the Aconitum State

Any condition that begins with the following unique combination of symptoms can be helped with *Aconitum*.

- Sudden onset
- Shock
- Fear, especially fear of death (usually for no reason)
- Restlessness
- Chill or extremely high fever (102F and above)

- Tremendous thirst
- Symptoms frequently begin after exposure to a chilling wind

Circumstances that trigger this combination of symptoms may include:

- Literally **any** acute condition accompanied by both severe fear (especially of imminent death) and restless anxiety.
- The very beginning of **colds**, **flu**, and **croup**, particularly when the onset is sudden and violent, or there is fear and agitation.
- Being a victim of, or witnessing, a horrific event. Interestingly, many people describe an event that provokes this state as a **"chilling experience."**

Aconitum states are usually brief. They're experienced, and witnessed by relatives and bystanders, in the first few minutes or hours after an event occurs or an acute illness sets in. After that, depending on how severe the reaction has been, it can either go away on its own (rare without homeopathy) or it can become worse—possibly leading to a more significant illness that requires treatment with heroic measures to save the person.

Common Colds and Flu

With rare exceptions, *Aconitum* is usually indicated in the first few hours (or even less) at the beginning of a severe head cold or flu. So, unless you get a chance to see a homeopath right away, you're going to need to take this remedy at home. After the initial stage is over, symptoms usually change and people therefore require a different remedy.

An additional clue that *Aconitum* is indicated is that people who need it commonly begin to feel worse late in the evening (twilight and later).

On several occasions, when my daughters were young, I had to give *Aconitum* to them or to the children of our neighbors at night, such as in the following case involving one of my daughters.

It was a nice, crispy cold November morning that was perhaps a bit too windy. My wife, our two children, and I went to see the Macy's Thanksgiving Day Parade and then we took a stroll around midtown Manhattan. Our children were dressed relatively well for the weather, however they took their hats off in the middle of our walk, insisting, for some reason, that wearing a winter hat was "not cool" (an interesting choice of words in such cold weather). The rest of the day was pleasant. We came home, had dinner with the family, and went to sleep early.

Around 11 PM, our elder daughter came to our bed saying that she felt very, very scared. She was shaking from chills. Soon after that, she developed a high fever and became increasingly frightened, anxious, and restless—all uncharacteristic for her. She said, "I've never been so scared in my life," yet couldn't explain why.

In order to make sure that I wasn't confusing my daughter's state with one that requires *Belladonna* (see Chapter 10), I looked into her eyes, and touched her head and hands. Her pupils were small, reflecting sheer horror, and her entire body was hot. She kept asking for additional glasses of cold water. If she had needed *Belladonna,* her hands and/or her feet would have been cold. Her pupils would have been so enlarged that she'd have looked as if she'd been drugged. Basically, she would look delirious, rather than agitated. Although she might have reported being scared, she wouldn't have been as restless as she was, and any fear would probably be linked to a scary dream or being afraid of the dark (ion other words, there would be some reason for it).

Now I knew! I gave my daughter a dose of three pellets of *Aconitum* 30C. She calmed down in five minutes or so, and went to sleep in another five to ten minutes. *That was it!* In the morning, she was completely recovered.

A skeptic might argue that my daughter would have gotten better anyway. But without homeopathy I don't believe her symptoms would have resolved as quickly as they did. If she'd recovered spontaneously, it's also unlikely there would have been no remnants of the previous night's symptoms whatsoever.

How is homeopathy better than Tylenol (acetaminophen) in such cases? After all, when you give a child a dose of Tylenol, his fever goes down and the child goes to sleep.

First, remember that you can always give someone Tylenol to suppress the symptoms of an illness after trying a homeopathic remedy. So, if it doesn't work you have another option. Certainly, when in doubt, you should *always* consult your physician or, if necessary, call 911. However, it is preferable to encourage the body's own sophisticated defense mechanisms to fight. If homeopathy does help someone improve, it means that person has done it on his own, and his immune system is being made stronger. A small dose of a natural substance does not mask symptoms.

Secondly, homeopathy produces no side effects. Interestingly, when high fevers are suppressed quickly with conventional medications, illness can continue to develop and the situation may become more serious despite (or due to) the lack of a general reaction. Fever serves a purpose in combating different illnesses.

Spending ten to fifteen minutes or less deciding upon a remedy, and another half an hour—maximum—waiting for the remedy you've chosen to work may save you and your family a lot of trouble and complications. But certainly, when you're in doubt, you should *always* consult your physician or, if necessary, call 911. Giving *Aconitum* to someone who is suffering on the way to the emergency room or doctor's office can make a dramatic difference in that person's life. If you, your child, or another family member improves after taking the remedy and therefore doesn't require dramatic, heroic treatments in the end, everybody will be happy.

Reminder: Aconitum is most frequently indicated at the first onset of an acute illness. If symptoms arise at night and you wait until the morning to select a remedy, another remedy should probably be used instead of *Aconitum.*

Let's briefly consider five other frequently indicated and easy-to-distinguish remedies.

Arsenicum album (arsenic trioxide): Used to treat influenza and colds that include gastroenteritis, vomiting, and diarrhea. Gastrointestinal complaints are usually prominent.

Please note: Unlike *Aconitum, Arsenicum* is indicated when there is a period of prodrome, or a gradual onset of symptoms.

Characteristic symptoms:
- High fever (up to 104 degrees) after a few-day onset. Fever may be followed by chill.
- Face is hot, the patient craves open air and cold applications to his head and face, yet the body is cold, chilled, and feels better from warmth.
- Thirsty for **small sips** of water (compare to *Bryonia* below).
- Significant restlessness with weakness and a tendency to collapse.
- Significant anxiety with fear of dying from this illness. Wants company at all times (compare with *Bryonia*).
- Worse: midnight or 1 AM, noon or 1 PM.

***Belladonna* (deadly nightshade):** Used for any type of acute illness (including colds and flu) that has a rapid onset and extremely high fever, especially if it's accompanied by delirious state. A commonly indicated remedy for children with high fever, the key indicator for *Belladonna* is a flushed red face that's hot to the touch, while hands and/or feet are cold.

Characteristic symptoms (also see Chapter 9):
- Almost delirious with possible hallucinations.
- Extremely high fevers (up to 105 degrees).
- Face is flushed.
- Pupils are dilated.
- Craves lemons and, frequently, lemonade.
- Frequently severe, right-sided headache (compare to *Bryonia* above).
- Headache is pounding. The person feels better in a dark, quiet room.
- Frequently right-sided sore throat or eye pain.
- Worse: frequently aggravated at 3 PM.

***Bryonia alba* (white bryony):** Used for slowly progressing influenza and common colds in which muscular aching is one of the important symptoms. The key indication is the desire to be absolutely still, as the patient feels much worse from the slightest movement. The patient does everything possible to save energy.

Characteristic symptoms:
- Feels restless internally, but cannot tolerate even the slightest motion.
- **Wants to be left alone**, doesn't want to answer questions, is irritable without expressing it aloud (compare with *Arsenicum*).

- Fever with the pronounced sensation of heat. Profuse perspiration.
- Chills begin distally (fingertips, toes, rarely the lips), and can be triggered by anger.
- Extremely thirsty for **large gulps** at intervals (compare to *Arsenicum* above).
- Severe headaches located on the front left side of the head or on the back of the head.
- Generally symptoms are worse on the right side of the body (except for the headache, which is left-sided).
- Worse: frequently at 9 PM, and **from the slightest motion.**
- Patients are usually warm and feel worse in warm rooms.

Eupatorium perfoliatum **(boneset):** Used for influenza that includes severe, unbearable aching. The key indicator is a terrible pain that feels as if the bones could break open.

Characteristic symptoms:
- High fever (usually over 102 degrees).
- Severe, unbearable aching.
- Chills begin in the area of the lower back and spread up the spine.
- Chills are worse after drinking.
- The patient is very chilly and sensitive to cold air.
- Thirsty for cold drinks despite the chill (and frequently during the chill).
- Desire for cold food and ice cream.
- Restless from the pain, but motion does not ameliorate.
- Worse: from 7 to 9 AM.

Table 8.1 Common Colds and Flu Remedy Comparison Chart

Remedy	Onset	Better	Worse
Aconitum	Sudden	Open air	Exposure to cold air, warm room; evening/ night, after midnight
Belladonna	Sudden	Lemonade; lemons	Afternoon, especially 3 PM
Arsenicum	Gradual	Company	Midnight or 1 PM
Bryonia	Slow progression	Being alone	Slightest movement; 9 PM
Eupatorium	Usually acute	Rest	Cold air; drinking (chills get worse); 7 to 9 AM
Gelsemium	Slow, over one to three days	Rest	Motion; 10 AM

Emotional State	Signs Guiding Your Selection	Reasons to Say No to This Remedy
Fearful; anxious; restless; children clingy with parents from fear	The very beginning of the illness; no discharges; small pupils; thirst for cold water; high fever and/or chills	Any discharge; late stages (more than a few hours) of illness; absence of fear or anxiety
Confused; possibly hallucinational; possibly appearing sedated	Flushed face; cold hands; dilated pupils; no thirst; frequently right-sided pounding headache	Small pupils; low-grade fever; significant thirst; discharges; late stages (more than 24 hours) of illness
Very anxious; frequently afraid to die from the illness	Hot face with the rest of the body being very cold; thirst for small sips of water; restlessness with weakness; frequently, diarrhea	Sudden onset; refuses company; thirst for very large amount of water
Wants to be left alone; refuses to answer questions; irritable	Tremendous thirst; fever with the sensation of heat and profuse perspiration; chills beginning from the fingertips and toes	Communicative; no thirst
Desperate and moaning from pain	Severe, unbearable aching; chills beginning in the lumbar region; and spreading up the spine; desire for cold food and drinks	No bone pains; no high fever; no chills
Very sleepy; depressed	Very heavy head, especially in the back; tremendous weakness with heaviness of the limbs and eyelids	Sudden onset; lack of weakness

Gelsemium sempervirens **(yellow jasmine):** Illness characterized by marked debility, weakness, and sleepiness. The onset is slow, lasting at least twenty-four hours to a few days. The key indicators are a heavy head, eyelids, and extremities and pronounced weakness with trembling.

Characteristic symptoms (also see Chapter 12, "Gelsemium"):
- **Head is very heavy, especially the back of the head.**
- Chills running up and down the spine.
- Chills that alternate with heat flushes.
- Chills accompanied by fine tremors.
- Minimal thirst.
- Extreme sleepiness.
- Eyelids are half shut or droopy.
- The patient is somewhat depressed, feels dull.
- Worse: aggravation at 10 AM.

Croup

Croup, the inflammation and narrowing of the air passages, is a potentially life-threatening early childhood illness that should be taken seriously by parents and guardians. Giving a child *Aconitum* can be A life-saving measure, as the following case, which took place more than fifty years ago, perfectly illustrates.

On a cold, dry winter day, when young Wayne was just under a year old, his parents took him out for a walk. It was quite windy. That night he woke up screaming. He had a high fever. His face was red when he was lying down, but turned pale when his parents picked him up. He also had a scary barking cough and his breathing was shallow. Each inhalation made him cough and suffocate even more. Drinking liquids made the cough worse. Wayne clung to his mother in fear.

Quickly realizing that their son had croup, his parents decided to go see an old German doctor who lived next door. The parents had known this kindly gentleman for many years and trusted his judgment. But still, his treatment seemed bizarre. The doctor examined Wayne, asked them some questions, and then gave their son a single pill. One little pill for a life-threatening situation? Seeing their concerned disbelief, the doctor asked them to wait patiently for a few minutes. Rapidly, in a matter of mere minutes, Wayne calmed down. Gradually his breathing became deeper. They took him home and put him to bed. He fell asleep in a matter of fifteen–twenty minutes more. When he woke up again a few hours later with a high fever, another little pill helped him to go back to sleep. In the morning Wayne was fine.

The German doctor was practicing homeopathy, so he knew to give Wayne *Aconitum* 30C in the early stage of croup. Wayne grew up to become a well-known integrative physician and today is one of my colleagues. He incorporates homeopathy in his medical practice. But he rarely sees cases of croup that require *Aconitum* for a simple reason: *Aconitum* is indicated in the first day, or even the first hour, of an attack. It should be given right at the onset, to stop the terror, on the way to the emergency room. Within a couple of hours, an untreated child would need another remedy.

We are living in the twenty-first century. There are no homeopathic doctors living next door to most American families—unless you're one of my neighbors. So parents must become familiar with signs indicating the need for *Aconitum* or a different remedy.

Characteristic indicators for *Aconitum* include:
- Sudden onset. Often begins after the exposure to cold, and most frequently to a combination of dry cold and wind.
- Fear and restlessness.

- The patient wakes up from the first part of sleep with a dry, barking, suffocating cough.
- Stridor, a shrill wheezing or grunting noise made by a child having difficulty breathing because the windpipe has become narrow.
- No mucous present.
- Child clings to parents.
- Worse: after each inhalation. Also when drinking (compare to *Spongia tosta* below).

It's also worth mentioning that children who require *Aconitum* for croup are usually robust, which is partly why they develop strong reactions to infections that include lots of heat and movement.

Table 8.2 Croup Remedy Comparison Chart

Remedy	Onset	Better	Worse
Aconitum	Sudden	Open air	Each inhalation; warm room; evening/night, after midnight
Spongia tosta	After *Aconitum*	Drinking/eating warm things; nursing; bending head forward; sitting upright	Cold drinks; talking; swallowing
Hepar sulphuris	After *Aconitum* and *Spongia*	Throwing head backward; eating	Slightest touch or draft; being uncovered

Here are two additional homeopathic remedies for croup.

Spongia tosta **(toasted sponge):** Probably the most frequently indicated remedy in the later stages (more than twenty-four hours after the onset) of croup. Essentially, if you don't see characteristic symptoms of *Aconitum, Spongia* should be your second possible choice.

Characteristic Symptoms:
- Dry, barking cough. Reminiscent of the sound of a saw going through wood. Some authors describe it as a "seal's bark."
- Stridor—the narrowing of the airways—with noisy, whistling sounds.
- Worse: at midnight or immediately after. Much worse from cold air or cold drinks.
- Better: after warm drinks or warm food. While eating, drinking, or nursing. While sitting upright or bent forward. Bending head forward (compare to *Hepar sulphuris calcareum* below).

Emotional State	Signs Guiding Your Selection	Reasons to Say No to This Remedy
Fearful; anxious; restless; children clingy with parents from fear	The very beginning of the illness; loud, difficult breathing; no mucous; high fever and/or chills	Any discharge; late stages (more than a few hours) of illness; absence of fear or anxiety
Anxious	Feeling cold; better from warm drinks; throat sensitive to touch	Worse from warm drinks or food; better from bending head backward
Very irritable and touchy; screams at the slightest provocation	Rattling mucous; very irritable	Better from bending head forward; no mucous

***Hepar sulphuris calcareum* (potassium salts):** The patient is irritable and touchy. Cannot tolerate even minimal discomfort. Might scream at the slightest provocation.

Characteristic symptoms:
- Croup comes on frequently between 2 and 4 AM or toward morning.
- Thick, rattling mucus.
- Worse: being uncovered, becoming even slightly cold.
- Better: Throwing the head backwards (compare to *Spongia tosta* above).

A note of caution: If a child or an adult is having difficulty breathing, you should seek immediate medical attention. A remedy (including *Aconitum*) should be given *on your way to the emergency room*. Don't lose precious time. You and your child are much better off wrong than sorry! In cases of croup, for example, a continuous wheezing breath could be a sign of a more serious problem—epiglottis—a serious illness that requires *immediate* professional attention.

Acute Post-Traumatic Stress Disorder

Nelly was a middle-aged woman who requested an immediate appointment to see me as she'd been mugged at gunpoint in the elevator of her apartment building the night before. After this terrorizing experience she had lost sleep. She found herself so scared that she couldn't lie down or even sit still. Thoughts of imminent death kept running through her mind. When one of her friends told Nelly about me, she wasted no time before phoning. She decided to see whether or not homeopathy could help her feel better.

The first thing I noticed when Nelly came into my office was an expression of fear on her face. She was terrified beyond an ability to function. A nice, polite person, she attempted to sit on the chair I offered, but was unable to remain still. Her legs, arms, and entire torso were continuously moving. I let her know that she didn't have to sit if she couldn't. While moving in circles around my small office, Nelly informed me that she was going to die soon. In fact, she was sure it was going to happen in exactly five days. She just "knew" it. Our interview was difficult. Nelly was obviously scared and anxious. She couldn't go on like that much longer. I quickly decided on the remedy: *Aconitum*.

Being an experienced homeopath I felt it was appropriate to give Nelly a dose of 200C. However, in your own "family practice," I recommend only using remedies in the homeopathic concentration 30C. The exception to this rule of thumb is *Arnica montana* (see Chapter 8).

The effect of the *Aconitum* was amazing. Literally, in three to five minutes after taking the dose Nelly was able to sit down. We continued our interview. By the time we finished (in another forty-five minutes or so), Nelly felt much better. I didn't give her any more remedies. That was it. For this most terrifying episode of her life, *Aconitum* did the job.

I see a lot of people with emotional problems in my practice, and I feel sorry when I find out that those who are suffering from post-traumatic stress didn't have access to *Aconitum* immediately after a horrifying experience. A significant proportion of people require *Aconitum* under those conditions. My friend Manfred, a homeopath from Germany, sent one kilogram (two pounds) of *Aconitum* to Honduras after a devastating earthquake. He travels there frequently and has been able to witness how much good *Aconitum* can do, when used judiciously.

Certainly, not every single individual who went through such an experience will need *Aconitum*. Many require another homeopathic remedy. In fact, even individuals who have had a similar experience may exhibit symptoms requiring different treatments.

Stramonium, another powerful homeopathic remedy has become one of the most important homeopathic remedies for treatment of post-traumatic stress disorder (PTSD). So important that I wrote a separate chapter about that remedy as, unfortunately, PTSD has become a part of life many individuals, families and a growing number of children.

A Few More Conditions That May Require Aconitum

There are many scenarios that may trigger *Aconitum* states, from experiencing an earthquake to being trapped in an enclosed space. A child who gets scared on an airplane and then runs around screaming from terror will generally do well after a dose of *Aconitum*, for example.

Some people are **morbidly afraid** of dentists. Imagine how wonderful it would be if anyone who feared death from pain could relax after taking a dose of *Aconitum*. Poor dental hygiene is a simple, everyday scenario that can lead to much worse conditions if it's left untreated. Resistant patients put themselves at risk when they avoid dental care. Likewise, a person who's avoiding necessary surgery due to dread and agitation may feel considerable relief from *Aconitum*.

A woman about to undergo a difficult labor who is feeling total panic and agitation could benefit from taking this remedy. So could a woman who's already given birth to a baby and is now bleeding, if her condition is accompanied by a tremendous fear of death, anxiety, and agitation.

Caution: While Aconitum *is generally safe for pregnant women and infants, if you are pregnant or nursing it is recommended to consult with a professional homeopath on the appropriate dosage before taking any remedies.*

A person who just sustained a significant physical injury and now feels restless and scared that he's going to die could also do well after the administration of *Aconitum*. The list of possible triggers mentioned here is only a guideline. Remember that homeopathy is used to treat individuals rather than specific illnesses or conditions.

When *Not* to Self-Medicate with *Aconitum*

- When the person is weak, and the reaction to the illness is also weak.
- When there is any kind of secretion (for example, significant amount of mucous in a child with croup). People who need *Aconitum* are usually dry and have no discharges. Remember that this remedy works well at the immediate onset of an illness. Discharges usually set in later.
- When there is no fear, anxiety, or agitation. With rare exception, **all** patients that require *Aconitum* show pronounced fear and restlessness.
- When faced with a chronic condition or a complex set of conditions.
- Although homeopathic remedies don't have side effects, when you are pregnant or breastfeeding the amount of time that you can safely spend trying to self-medicate with various remedies is significantly less, so please seek the advice of a health care professional immediately.

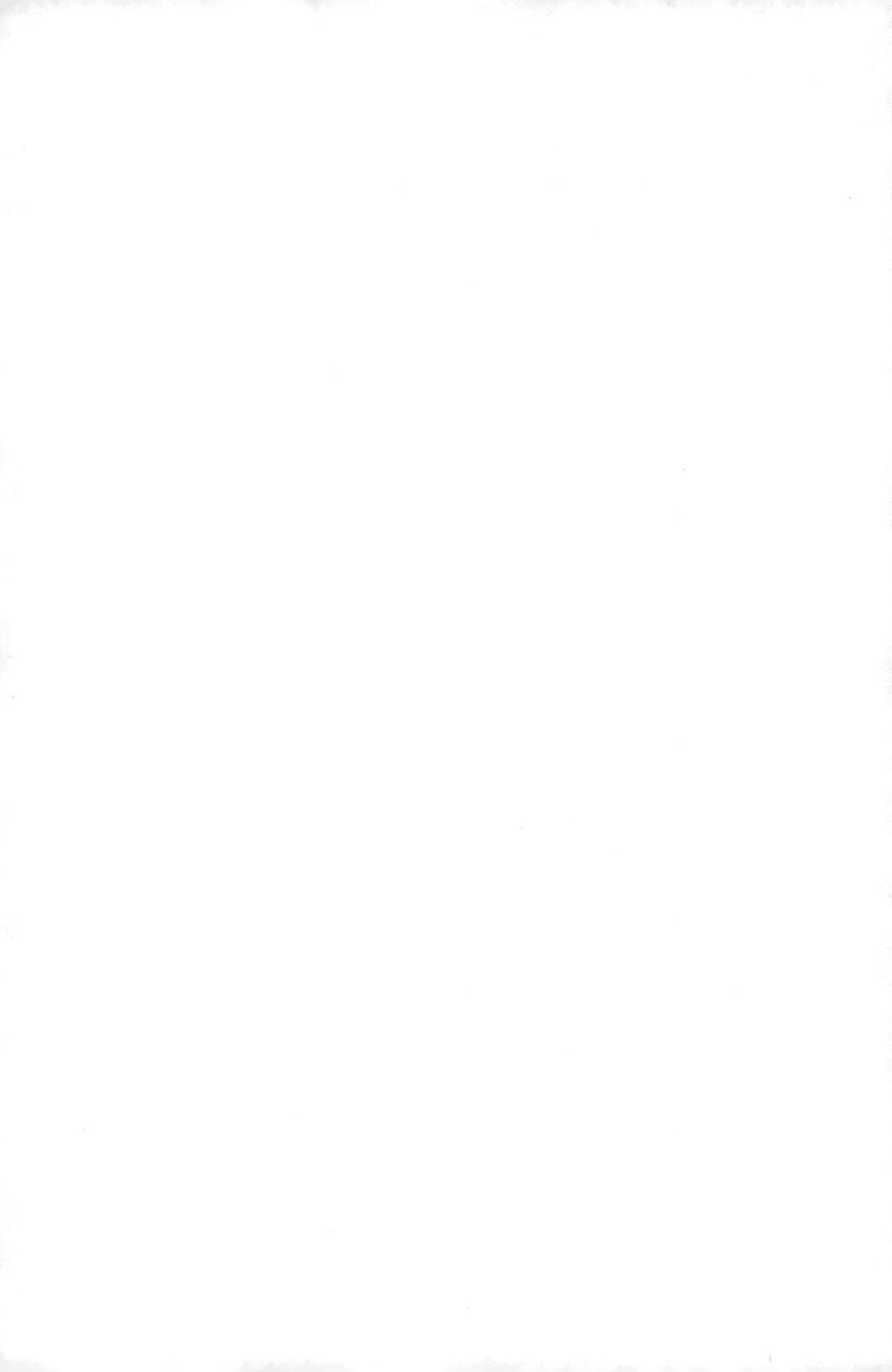

CHAPTER NINE

Arnica
Your Homeopathic Surgeon

*"Children show scars like medals.
Lovers use them as secrets to reveal."*
—LEONARD COHEN

The healing properties of **Arnica montana (leopard's bane),** the second in our growing collection of outstanding remedies, have been recognized for millennia. Well known to the ancient Greeks and Romans for its medicinal powers to heal **wounds** and **falls,** in antiquity they called the plant *Panacea lapsorum,* literally meaning "cure for falls." As you can see from this brief history, Arnica—even the nonhomeopathic herb—has long been celebrated as a remedy par excellence for the treatment of **injuries.**

Samuel Hahnemann already possessed many good sources of information when he decided to conduct provings of this important plant. His research confirmed the herb's amazing curative properties and revealed many characteristics unique to patients needing Arnica. Interestingly, the majority of victims of the kind of trauma where the major impact is on the muscles and bones develop symptoms calling for this seemingly magical remedy. In his description of *Arnica,*

Hahnemann wrote: "The symptoms of all injuries caused by severe contusions and lacerations of the fibers [*muscles—author*] are tolerably uniform in character, and . . . these symptoms are contained in striking homoeopathic similarity in the alterations of the health which arnica develops in the healthy human subject."[1]

This chapter will explore the uses of *Arnica* and other remedies beneficial for treating general injuries and trauma, eyes injuries in specific, postoperative recovery, bites and insect stings, burns, near drowning, and fainting. As you'll discover, *Arnica* is an incredibly valuable item to keep stocked in your home medicine cabinet.

The Origins of *Arnica*

Leopard's bane, the folk name for our herb, reflects the similarity of its bright yellow flowers to the eyes of a wildcat. The name *Arnica* is derived from the Greek word for lamb, *arnos,* which refers to the similarity in texture of its leaves and flowers to the soft fur of the farm animal. *Montana* signals that the plant grows at high altitudes.

Mountain dwellers understood the therapeutic qualities of the herb, which conveniently grows in the mountains of Germany, Switzerland, and Siberia, and they used its infusion to cure ailments related to falls and head trauma. (An infusion is a solution made by steeping an herb in water.) Legend has it that in olden times mountain climbers chewed fresh leaves from the plant to ease the soreness of their muscles and to help their bruises heal faster. But, as we know today, raw *Arnica* is poisonous.

Warning: You should never ingest the Arnica plant itself. Only homeopathically prepared Arnica *is safe for consumption.*

In German folk medicine arnica was called *fallkraut* (fall weed). Hildegard of Bingen, the illustrious German nun—a visionary, composer, and accomplished naturalist and herbal healer, whom the Catholic Church has beatified—wrote extensively about the properties of arnica in the beginning of the twelfth century.[2]

Homeopathic *Arnica montana* is prepared from the whole fresh plant when it is in bloom. Its preparations have been successfully used for the effective and extremely prompt treatment of both severe and mild injuries, and in the prevention of complications from surgery. That's why *Arnica* is a cornerstone of homeopathic first aid. If you could remember only a single homeopathic remedy, *Arnica* would be that remedy, as it helps so many children and adults avoid potential complications of severe trauma. It saves lives.

In many ways *Arnica* has become a symbol of homeopathy. Most health food stores now carry it in gels and ointments, as well as standard pellets. Nearly all parents in large industrial centers know something about *Arnica*, and use it to handle everything that comes up in their households from minor bruises to cases of severe trauma.

Symptoms Characteristic of the Arnica State

As repeatedly mentioned, *Arnica* is the main remedy indicated in cases of trauma. It is so effective in this regard, in fact, that some homeopathic authors have compared similarly valuable remedies for other types of conditions to it. For instance, you may read, "*Ignatia* is *Arnica* for the emotions." Although it is true that cases of severe trauma and surgical interventions producing damage to both muscles and superficial bone structures almost always require this remedy, it is also true that there are highly specific emotional symptoms and modalities that pinpoint the need (or lack thereof) for Arnica. As you'll recall, a modality is something that makes a condition better or worse.[3]

If you or someone else in your family is exhibiting the correct physical, mental, and emotional indicators, *Arnica* is the remedy for the condition you are treating. If not, then taking another remedy is more appropriate.

Once you've identified that it is the appropriate remedy, *Arnica* must be administered in a particular dose and following a particular schedule. Mindless use of *Arnica* for minor bruises, or unnecessary repetitions of *Arnica* before and after surgery may lead someone who consumes it to experience certain complications, such as bruising. As you already understand from reading Chapter 3, too frequent administration of a single homeopathic remedy can exacerbate your symptoms for the same reasons that the remedy could cause a proving in a healthy, sensitive individual.

Later in this chapter, I'll give you detailed instructions for administering *Arnica*.

The most characteristic symptoms of *Arnica* are:
- A sore, bruised feeling.
- Feeling beaten, either in the entire body or in the affected part.
- Restlessness in bed because it feels too hard.
- Shock after injury, the person often denies needing help or that anything is wrong.
- Fear after accidents.
- Bleeding (for example, a nosebleed) after washing the face. Renowned American homeopath Paul Herscu has described how he used *Arnica* to cure a pregnant woman who developed uterine bleeding after washing her face.

Things that make the condition feel worse include:
- Touch: The person in this state frequently does not allow themself to be touched.
- Heat.
- Rest on one side, or being in one position for too long.
- At night, after sleep.

Things that make the condition feel better include:
- Lying down with head low—flat on your back.
- Cold applications.
- Open air.
- Changing position.

Circumstances that often require using *Arnica* as the first choice:
- Any **severe accident** that would require you to call 911.
- **Trauma:** first remedy for injuries of soft tissues (skin plus muscle), such as injuries from blows, falls, or strikes from blunt objects
- Concussion of the brain (after jarring head injuries and motor vehicle accidents). Headache, dizziness, personality changes, memory loss, or feeling foggy, distracted, or fatigued are all subtle symptoms of this condition.
- Bleeding caused by injury.
- Shock from injury.
- Fear after injury.
- Soreness after tooth extraction or dental surgery.
- Prophylactically, before dental or other surgery, when you know there is going to be damage to skin, muscle, and bone (for example, during wisdom tooth extraction, or any other serious dental surgery, orthopedic surgery, facial plastic surgery, breast augmentation, and mastectomy)

Injuries and Trauma

The rule of thumb is the sooner you give *Arnica,* the better. Personally, I always carry *Arnica montana* 10M in the glove compartment of my car in case I happen to pass a serious motor vehicle accident along the road I'm driving.

In an emergency, give an accident victim three pellets of *Arnica montana* 200C (or 1M, 10M, or 50M) on the way to the emergency room. Usually these doses are sufficient for moderate to serious injuries. For minor injuries, or if you do not have any other potency on hand, you can use 30C tablets. Give the accident victim three pellets under the tongue right away and follow with two to three more doses at fifteen- to thirty-minute intervals.

Here are a couple of additional principles to keep in mind.

- The more severe an injury is, the higher the potency of *Arnica* you should use, and the less time there should be between repetitions.
- I strongly recommend that you don't exceed three repetitions. The only exception would be when the trauma is severe but only *Arnica montana* 30C is available. In that case you should repeat the dose every fifteen minutes for up to five times.

Hahnemann suggested simultaneous external and internal use of *Arnica* in cases where there is damage to the skin and/or muscles.

For minor injuries, such as superficial bruises and bumps, apply an *Arnica* gel or ointment topically on the skin. There is no reason to take *Arnica* pills in such cases, as no actual damage has been done. The body of the injured person, especially if it is a healthy child, should be able to deal with minor problems without unnecessary help. Parents too frequently give their children *Arnica* tablets for minor bruises. This is a mistake, as the use of *Arnica* ointment alone is effective.

Warning: Do not use Arnica *gels and ointments if the skin is broken, as it is an irritant.*

One of my adult patients suffered significant bruising after a car accident. Her family members knew the benefits of *Arnica,* yet they only had *Arnica* ointment on hand. Her sister applied the ointment everywhere on her body that they could see was already developing a bruise. Interestingly, in a few days the treated areas had no bruising, while the areas that were ignored, because they originally had no obvious bruising, turned black and blue. In this situation, *Arnica montana* 200C tablets would also have been appropriate.

I can recall plenty of situations where *Arnica* was clearly indicated and prevented extremely serious complications. The two that follow involved experienced homeopaths.

In the first case, a well-known homeopathic teacher was walking back into the classroom after a break. Because he was thoroughly engaged in an animated conversation with one of his students he literally walked into the doorframe at a pretty good speed. The impact was significant. The man almost fell and looked confused for a brief moment. Quickly he then stated, "I'm OK guys. I need no help." Even before the end of this phrase the entire class and the teacher himself started to laugh. We all recognized his statement as one of the main characteristics of the *Arnica* state: he believed he was OK despite experiencing a severe blow. Fortunately a few people in class had homeopathic kits with them containing *Arnica.* The teacher's head and our schedule were both saved.

Another scary scenario unfolded on Alonissos, a beautiful Greek island that is famous in homeopathic circles since it houses the International Academy of Homeopathy run by the world renowned homeopath George Vithoulkas. Several years ago I arrived there to conduct a small research study with a large group of experienced homeopaths and was invited for a "safe" boat trip to get to know them. I do get seasick easily, but I was told that we would just eat, have a few drinks, watch the stars, and socialize. And the promise was made that the sea would be quiet that evening, so of course a storm set in right in the middle of our trip and knocked someone over. I saw the accident happen because I was sitting in the stern of the boat turning green from nausea and trying to get as much air as I could.

As a wave rocked the boat, one of my fellow homeopaths slipped on the floor and hit a bench with the back of his head. We all heard a scary sound from the impact of his head against the wood of the bench. A few people surrounded the man. Although he was bleeding, the first words out of his mouth were, "I'm OK, guys. No big deal!" You can be sure he received *Arnica* almost immediately and that the dose was repeated a few times.

To the total surprise and utter disbelief of many medical staffs, on some occasions the victim of a serious accident will arrive at the ER without showing signs of the typical pain and swelling, because they've taken a few doses of *Arnica*. Of course, a fracture always requires prompt professional intervention so bones can be set and complications prevented. However, the amount of pain and swelling accompanying a fracture, if you take *Arnica,* is usually significantly less than otherwise expected in such a severe case.

Here are ten other remedies that may be indicated for accident victims. *Please note:* Eye injuries will be separately discussed in the next section, as there are so many different possible remedies from which to choose.

***Aconitum napellus* (monkshood):** Usually indicated in the first moments after a horrific trauma when someone becomes morbidly scared with severe agitation and restlessness (also see Chapter 8, "Aconitum").

- Sudden onset
- Shock
- Fright
- Fear, especially fear of death (usually for no reason)
- Restlessness
- Chill or extremely high fever
- Tremendous thirst
- Symptoms frequently begin after exposure to chilling wind

***Bellis perennis* (common daisy):** Indicated for cases of trauma to internal organs, such as the liver, spleen, or uterus. It is also appropriate if swelling persists for a long time after an injury, despite administering *Arnica* or another appropriate remedy.

***Bryonia alba* (white bryony):** Seriously consider this remedy whenever trauma to the bones is involved. You can recognize this because the victim will refuse to move.

- **Severe pain and discomfort made worse by even the slightest motion**
- Feels restless internally, but cannot tolerate even the slightest motion
- **Wants to be left alone,** doesn't want to answer questions, is irritable without expressing it aloud
- Better: from anything that prevents motion, such as firm pressure or lying on the injured part of the body

***Carbo vegetabilis* (vegetable charcoal):** Indicated when the victim faints.
- Needs constant fanning
- Severe weakness
- Significant coldness of the injured area

***Chamomilla* (German chamomile):** Indicated for fainting from severe pain.
- Extremely sensitive to pain
- Better and worse: no specific modalities in this situation; the patient just needs *Chamomilla* to get better.

***Ferrum phosphoricum* (phosphate of iron).**
This remedy is good for:
- Fever after a head injury.
- Better: cold applications.
- Worse: at night and 4–6 AM; also from touch, jarring, and motion.

***Hamamelis virginiana* (witch hazel):** *Instructions*: To increase its action against bruising, try combining *Hamamelis* ointment or gel with an equal amount of *Arnica* ointment. Apply twice a day. The person in this state has:
- Severe bruises that swell and bleed.
- Nosebleeds that last a long time, even after you give *Arnica*.

***Hypericum perforatum* (St. John's wort):** Appropriate for trauma to parts of the body reached by peripheral nerves, such as crushed fingers and toes, and spinal injuries.
- The person may be depressed or upset after injury
- Better: from rubbing and rest

- Worse: from cold, foggy weather, and dampness

Ruta graveolens **(garden rue):** This remedy is useful for trauma to the periosteum (connective tissue that wraps around the bones), especially in areas where the bone is close to the skin, like the shinbone, the pelvis, and the elbow. The person who needs it is:
- Restless because of soreness.
- Anxious, irritable, and upset with others.
- Better: from continuous, gentle motion.
- Worse: from first motion, sitting, and touch.

Sanguinaria canadensis **(bloodroot):** Almost a specific remedy for post-traumatic **right shoulder** pain. (Sorry, homeopaths don't have a similar remedy yet for the left shoulder!)

Instructions: Take three pellets of *Sanguinaria canadensis* 12C once a day for twenty days. Stop taking doses if your pain disappears earlier.
- The person in this state is irritable in the evening, wants to be held and comforted.
- Better: from rest and lying down.
- Worse: at night and from raising the arm.

Symphytum officinale **(comfrey):** An excellent remedy for nonunion of the bones.

Instructions: Take five pellets of *Symphytum officinale* 6C three times a day for twenty days—or fewer days in cases of a speedy recovery.

Table 9.1 Injuries and Trauma Remedy Comparison Chart

Type of Trauma	Remedy	Better	Worse
The main remedy to consider for any physical trauma	*Arnica*	Cold applications; lying down, especially with head low; changing position	Touch; jarring; drinking wine
Initial stages of any trauma, physical and emotional	*Aconitum*	No specific factors; generally better in the open air	Lying on the painful side; warm room
Trauma to internal organs (liver, spleen, uterus); swelling that does not go away after *Arnica*	*Bellis*	Continued motion; rest; cold applied locally	Chill and being wet; hot bathing and warmth of bed; before storm
Any acute trauma with typical symptoms, especially trauma to the bones and joints	*Bryonia*	Immobilization of injured part, from lying on painful side, a brace, a tight bandage, pressure; local heat	Any motion, even turning slightly, moving the eyes, or taking a deep breath
Fainting after severe injury	*Carbo vegetabilis*	Desire to be fanned	No modalities related to trauma
Fainting from pain	*Chamomilla*	No specific modalities in this particular case	Severe pain, as perceived by the victim

Emotional State	Signs Guiding Your Selection	Reasons to Say No to This Remedy
In shock after injury; convinced nothing is wrong; sends help away	First remedy for blunt injury, bruising, accidents; thoughts that everything is OK, despite sometimes having severe injury; inability to find comfortable position in bed because it feels too hard	In cases of broken skin (open wounds) do not use ointment or tincture
Fearful, anxious, and restless, frequently with fear of imminent death	Extreme fear with restlessness immediately after trauma	Absence of fear or anxiety
No specific mental picture has been described yet	Intense soreness; trauma to internal organs; after *Arnica* failed	Rarely indicated as the first remedy after musculoskeletal trauma (start from *Arnica*)
Very irritable and touchy; screams at the slightest provocation; wants to be alone (due to fear of being touched)	Much worse from motion; trauma to bone structures; does not want to be disturbed	Moves without problems, or with pain, but does not require to be absolutely still
No modalities related to trauma	Desire to be fanned	Fainting from severe pain (instead give *Chamomilla*); no fainting; no need for constant fanning
No modalities related to trauma	Extreme sensitivity to slightest pain	When symptoms clearly indicate *Carbo vegetabilis*

Table 9.1 Injuries and Trauma Remedy Comparison Chart *(continued)*

Type of Trauma	Remedy	Better	Worse
Fever after head injury	***Ferrum phosphoricum***	Cold applications	At night and 4 to 6 AM; touch; jarring; motion
Severe bruises that swell and bleed even after *Arnica*	***Hamamelis***	No modalities related to trauma	No modalities related to trauma
Crushed fingers and/or toes; spinal injury; injury to peripheral nerves	***Hypericum***	Rubbing; rest	Cold; cold, foggy weather; dampness
Trauma to tendons; trauma to wrist, shin, knee, ankle	***Ruta***	Continued gentle motion	First motion; sitting; touch
Right-sided post-traumatic shoulder pain	***Sanguinaria***	Rest; lying down	Raising the arm; at night
Fracture; non-union of bones	***Symphytum***	No specific modalities	No specific modalities

Emotional State	Signs Guiding Your Selection	Reasons to Say No to This Remedy
No modalities related to trauma	Fever after head injury with few or no modalities; no typical modalities for *Arnica* or other remedies described	Lack of fever (in that case, give *Arnica*)
No specific trauma-related symptoms	Large, swollen, bleeding bruises that remain after *Arnica*	No significant bruising prior to use of *Arnica*
May be depressed or upset after injury; rarely may report that after injury head feels longer or even lifted in the air	Crushed fingers; trauma to peripheral nerves and spine	Significant trauma to peripheral nerves and/or fingers or toes
Restless because of soreness; anxious; irritable; upset with others	For trauma to the wrist and periosteum	No significant trauma to periosteum or wrist
Irritable in the evening; wants to be held and comforted	Specific for right-sided shoulder trauma (chronic or acute)	Left-sided complaints
No specific modalities	Fractures; nonunion of bones	Bones not yet set by a specialist

Eye Injuries

Our eyes are some of the most sensitive territory in our bodies and need to be protected. Before covering any other topics, if there is a speck in the eye, be aware that it must be removed by being flushed out with liquid. *Warning: Never touch an eye with anything dry.* In case of emergency when you don't have access to homeopathy use a mild saline solution designed for rinsing out contact lenses. Otherwise use the following solution.

To flush a speck out of your own or someone else's eye, add half a teaspoon of a homeopathically prepared *Calendula officinalis* tincture to a cup of cold water, and then use this mixture as eyewash. (A tincture is an alcohol-based solution.) You could also use this mixture to relieve irritation and pain after the removal of a foreign body in the eye.

Please remember that we live in the twenty-first century and eye doctors are easy to locate. Go see one if the need arises. Better safe than sorry.

Now, *Arnica* is effective if someone gets a black eye after walking into a door, or from receiving a blow above or below the eye. Other remedies may be better for handling different types of eye injuries, such as inflammation, irritation, hemorrhages, and so on.

Let's evaluate some of the most commonly required options. In this particular case there is no time or need to belabor modalities or other symptoms. All that's important for your decision-making process information is presented below in a very few sentences.

Aconitum napellus **(monkshood):** Old-time homeopaths used to call this remedy "*Arnica montana* of the eye." It relieves pain and inflammation. Be aware, you might feel temporary relief even if a speck is still in your eye, then the pain will come back until it's ultimately removed. If children won't allow you to open their eyes and look for a speck, give *Aconitum* and bring them to the eye doctor or the ER.

Calendula officinalis **(marigold):** To treat bleeding for a cut eyelid, soak a gauze pad in a mixture of half a teaspoon of *Calendula* tincture and a cup of cold water, and then apply the pad to the cut with gentle pressure.

Hamamelis virginiana **(witch hazel):** A specific remedy for traumatic bleeding inside the eye.

Hypericum perforatum **(St. John's wort):** Give one dose of 30C internally for severe pain in the eye after the injury. You can also prepare eyewash from *Hypericum* tincture (use similar proportions to *Calendula officinalis* above) and use it externally.

Ledum palustre **(marsh tea):** Beneficial for a black eye that feels much better from cold applications.

Symphytum officinalis **(comfrey):** The main remedy for blows directly to the eyeball; it is also useful in relieving long-lasting pain or soreness after an eye injury.

Surgery, Before and After

As I stated before, giving people too much *Arnica* can cause provings in them. Plastic surgeons and individuals who undergo plastic surgery have known about the benefits of homeopathic *Arnica* for a long time. But some surgeons got so excited about its effects that they suggested that their patients take it for two weeks prior to surgery and then take additional postoperative doses. To their surprise, patients were more bruised and bled more than normal. These complications clearly resulted from misuse.

A simple schedule is to take three pellets of *Arnica* 200C right before surgery, three pellets after the surgery is finished (if dental surgery is being done under local anesthesia, ask your dentist to place three pellets in your mouth) or after you wake up from anesthesia; and three pellets that night before going to sleep.

Here are five remedies that people undergoing surgery often benefit from taking instead of *Arnica*. As you can see, the instructions below are simple and straightforward, without bulleted entries. Usually the few symptoms listed below will suffice to give you a good idea about what remedy to choose.

***Aconitum napellus* (monkshood):** This remedy is helpful for shock and fright before and after surgery when the person is morbidly scared and—especially—convinced that he or she will die during the operation.

Instructions: One to two doses of 30C or 200C every fifteen minutes can make a huge difference. (Compare with *Gelsemium* below.)

***Calendula officinalis* (marigold):** This remedy helps to speed up the healing of surgical wounds without complications.

Instructions: The most efficient way to use it is to take five pellets of *Calendula officinalis* 6C three times a day for twenty days, and also to apply *Calendula* ointment on the wound (after the surgeon removes the dressing) twice a day.

***Gelsemium sempervirens* (yellow jasmine):** This remedy works well for severe anxiety before surgery. The individual in this state may be trembling with fear and feels weak. Compare the picture for *Gelsemium* with the *Aconitum* state, where a reaction is strong, and includes terror and overwhelming fear of death. (Also see Chapter 12, "Gelsemium.")

Phosphorus **(phosphorus):** This remedy helps relieve bad effects of anesthesia, like disorientation, anxiety, nausea, and vomiting. It's helpful for nausea and vomiting after abdominal surgery. The most characteristic symptom in these cases is vomiting immediately after food or drinks warm up in stomach (usually a few minutes after ingestion).

Staphysagria **(staph):** This remedy helps in cases of trauma and/or pain and even bleeding after urinary catheterizations.
Instructions: Take three pellets of *Staphysagria* 30C three times at fifteen-minute intervals on your way to the urologist. In cases where there are complications you should always consult a physician. Better safe than sorry.

Bites and Insect Stings

An animal bite (or human bite) or insect sting can pose an emergency. When you are faced with these kinds of trauma, *Arnica* is a possibility, but it is not the first solution you should be considering.

Most often, insect stings and bites *don't* require any kind of treatment other than cleaning out the wound with soap and water. Hydrogen peroxide is always a good choice, too, as it kills many dangerous bacteria and cleans wounds well. But as they do after their children take minor falls, parents frequently overuse homeopathic remedies in cases of insect bites, even though an uncomplicated sting from one bee doesn't require a remedy.

My favorite external application for beestings is a product called Gold Star balm, which is sold in Chinese and Korean stores. It comes in a cute little red tin container with, as you might imagine, a gold star on it. A single application usually takes the itching and stinging sensation away and reduces localized swelling. If you don't have a balm handy, ice and a little bit of aloe vera would probably solve the problem.

Now, if someone has a systemic reaction to an insect bite or sting, and/or if the area becomes significantly swollen and painful, a homeopathic remedy can do miracles.

Animal bites and human bites present significant problems, as they get infected quickly and have a tendency to heal slowly with a lot of complications. Homeopathic remedies promote faster healing of such injuries, and decrease or sometimes even prevent scar formation. The sooner someone gets the right remedy, the better the outcome will be.

Please don't forget to clean and disinfect bite wounds, too.

Here are very helpful remedies for different kinds of bites and stings. As you'll notice from the following descriptions, *Arnica* cannot be considered a primary remedy for these conditions. But one can never rule it out entirely.

The remedies are listed in the alphabetic order, but the main remedy for small insect stings and bites that you should always consider first is *Apis mellifica*. For stings and bites of larger insects such as wasps give a strong consideration to *Ledum pallustre*.

The remedy t consider first for animal bites is also *Ledum*.

For bites of venomous snakes, first think about *Lachesis mutus*.

Arnica montana (leopard's bane): *Arnica* is appropriate for bites whenever you see significant trauma to a combination of skin, muscles, and even a bone. The only other possible situation is a bite by a large dog without any damage done to the skin. Typically for the *Arnica* state, the victim will not consider the situation serious.

Aconitum napellus (monkshood): I've seen cases when a child, or even an adult, stung by a bee gets so scared that the need for *Aconitum* is obvious. Use it if someone is scared, red-faced, and has an expression of terror such that the pupils of the eyes become tiny. One dose of *Aconitum* 30C will resolve this issue, and then you have to wait and see. Taking this remedy may be sufficient, or afterward the victim may also develop symptoms that indicate a need for another remedy listed below.

Apis mellifica (honey bee): This is the main remedy for insect stings and bites. Use this remedy if the area of a sting is swollen red, **warm to the touch,** and the condition is made better by cold. (Compare the person's symptoms with the picture of *Ledum* in which the area is usually cold and reddish-blue.) Frequently, the person who needs *Apis* is quite irritable; it's easy for this individual to "fly off the handle." I've seen cases of severe allergic reactions to beestings that almost instantly respond to *Apis*. Severe swelling with inflammation after stings from other insects responds similarly well.

Instructions: A dose of 30C is good, either dry or in water (for example, the plussing method, see Chapter 3). If there's an initial, but not a complete improvement, repeat the dose two more times at thirty- to sixty-minute intervals. Stop giving doses sooner if the victim is more than 50 percent better.

Don't use *Apis,* or any other remedy for that matter, just because there's a situation in which it's frequently indicated. Frequently, the bites of wasps and other large insects require *Ledum palustre*—but not always. Assess what's going on with the victim for a few minutes before making your selection.

***Ledum palustre* (marsh tea):** This remedy is almost a specific for animal bites, including those from dogs, cats, raccoons, and snakes, and human bites, and for the stings and bites of large insects, such as wasps. A main indication is that the area of the bite or sting is reddish-blue and surrounded by a very pale area. The wound is also **cold to the touch** (compare with *Apis mellifica*). This remedy is appropriate for puncture wounds and bites—both human and animal.

Paradoxically, ice-cold applications bring about a dramatic improvement although the areas of the bite are cold. In this picture, the patient won't let go of the icepack! (Compare with the picture of *Arsenicum* in which the area is hot, and the pain is improved by hot applications. If that happens and the patient is anxious, *Arsenicum* should be your first choice).

***Urtica urens* (stinging nettle):** For stings of jellyfish and medusa. Also use for any other type of insect bites or stings in which the main symptoms are hives and itching that get better from rubbing the area. Some people in need for this remedy simply cannot stop rubbing the wound.

Scorpions, Snakes, and Spider Bites and Severe Reactions

Homeopathy is effective in the treatment of bites by scorpions, snakes, and spiders. It's also effective for treatment of severe allergic reactions to bites and stings, including anaphylactic shock. Below please find a description of a few remedies that can be helpful with these issues. If you're an avid traveler and your family spends time in the wilderness, make sure you have these remedies handy, along with other first-aid items.

Carbolicum acidum **(carbolic acid):** A remedy of choice for severe allergic reactions to beestings, insect bites, and animal bites, it's also useful for anaphylaxis. In this picture the patient has a dusky red face, but the skin around the mouth and nose is pale. The victim also reports a choking feeling and frequently becomes lethargic, but, even so, may paradoxically develop an acute awareness of odors. In cases of allergic reactions, someone develops hives over the entire body.

Instructions: Give repeated 30C doses every ten to fifteen minutes until improvement or the arrival of the ambulance. You should *always* call 911 or go to the ER if you see these symptoms develop. If the condition arises during a camping trip, give the remedy and head towards a populated area as fast as you can!

Lachesis muta **(bushmaster snake venom):** Constantine Hering discovered this important homeopathic remedy over one hundred years ago. In cases of poisonous bites by snakes or spiders, it can be beneficial. The affected part has a dusky, purple color. Frequently, you'll see a continuous oozing of blood from the wound.

Instructions: Give a 200C dose once and apply an icepack to prevent the poison from spreading. Of course, professional help *must* be on its way or you should be rushing towards the nearest hospital *right away!*

Oxalicum acidum **(oxalic acid):** This remedy works well if the affected part becomes numb and cold to the touch, and the victim also reports violent pains and begins to tremble. It's imperative to rush the victim to the nearest hospital! Give one dose of the remedy on your way.

Table 9.2 Bites and Insect Stings Remedy Comparison Chart

Type of Trauma	Remedy	Better	Worse
Psychological trauma immediately after the bite or even at the sight of an animal or insect (humans bite too)	*Aconitum*	No specific modalities	No specific modalities
Bee and other small animal stings	*Apis*	Cold applications	Heat locally and generally
Wasps and other large insect bites; remedy of choice for tick bites; remedy of choice for animal/human bites	*Ledum*	Ice-cold applications	Heat, although the person is chilly; even the slightest touch or pressure
Jellyfish and medusa stings; insect bites and stings	*Urtica urens*	Continuous rubbing	No specific modalities
Severe allergic reaction to bee and other insect stings and bites	*Carbolicum acidum*	No specific modalities	No specific modalities
Poisonous bites by snakes/large spiders	*Lachesis*	No specific modalities	Heat
Severe reactions to snake bites	*Oxalicum acidum*	No specific modalities	Thinking about the problem; touch; light

Emotional State	Signs Guiding Your Selection	Reasons to Say No to This Remedy
Fearful (frequently fearful of imminent death); anxious; restless	Extreme fear (including fear of dying); panic; restlessness; immediately after a bite	Absence of fear and anxiety
Irritable; busy	Stinging (like from a bee sting) pain; swelling; redness; area is warm or hot to touch	Absence of swelling with redness and heat
Wants to be alone	Bite area is cold to touch; person is cold but wants ice-cold applications to the wound and won't let go of it; bite area is bluish	Feeling of heat; irritability
No specific modalities	Blotches (urticaria) with violent itching (like from stinging nettles); gets better from constant rubbing	No blotches
Lethargic	Severe allergic reactions to bee stings (could be to other insects) with dusky face, but skin around mouth and nose is pale; blotches and/or vesicles covering entire body	Agitation and irritability (think about *Apis*)
Anxious	Dusky purple bite area with oozing blood	No obvious signs to say no
Confused; feels worse thinking about the problem	Numbness; violent pain; trembling	Needs to be rushed to the nearest hospital

Burns

In December 2002, famous homeopaths Roger Morrison, M.D., and Nancy Herrick, P.A., happened to be in Bali during a terrorist bombing that caused massive damage and killed hundreds of people. Rushing to the local hospital to help, they discovered a scene of utter chaos.

Reporting in a *Homeopathy Today* article, Morrison explains that the majority of injuries were burns. "Nancy and I spent the first six hours debriding burns and changing dressings. Luckily we had a few homeopathic remedies with us—including *Arnica* and *Aconite* 200C, known for their effectiveness in cases of trauma and shock. It is a rare opportunity to see homeopathy working in cases so extreme, and the results in cases of shock were astonishing even to us. People who were lying paralyzed with fixed gaze began sitting up and speaking minutes after the remedy."[4]

Serious burns always have to be treated in a hospital setting. Burn victims may require intravenous fluids, pain medication, antibiotics, and other supplies. You shouldn't delay seeking professional medical attention in order to select the right remedy. Rush the burn victim to the hospital and give the best remedy you can on the route there.

For minor burns, Hahnemann advised using warm applications, a practice which makes sense homeopathically. Of course, the majority of burn victims ask to be given cold applications. Folk medicine also recommends touching your own earlobe in cases of minor burns to the fingertips, as the earlobe is usually cold.

After cleaning the burned area and making sure it is dry, apply homeopathically prepared *Calendula* ointment or lotion. Then, if the picture of the remedy's characteristic symptoms seems appropriate, give the person who's been burned one of these remedies. Do not apply anything except for covering the area with dry sterile gauze if the burned area has blisters or boils. In this case, seek professional help immediately!

Apis mellifica **(honey bee):** For minor burns that are greatly relieved by ice-cold applications, and which are red and swollen. This remedy is also helpful for treating chemical burns to the eyes.

Caution: If you don't know how to handle chemical burns, don't interfere with the efforts of trained professionals or a first-response team.

Arsenicum album **(oxide of arsenic):** This remedy is beneficial for severe burns (third degree), and for burns accompanied by significant anxiety and restlessness. Note that the victim refuses cold applications and feels better from warm applications.

Cantharis **(Spanish fly):** Usually used for second-degree and third-degree burns with extreme burning pain. Unlike *Arsenicum,* this victim desire ice-cold applications. The person simply wouldn't let go of an icepack. It works for chemical burns, too.

Note: A prompt administration of this remedy may prevent the formation of blisters.

Urtica urens **(stinging nettle):** Beneficial for minor burns caused by scalding hot boiling water.
Furthermore, if the victim is terrified by the traumatic experience of being burned, it is appropriate to give *Aconitum* instead of *Arnica*.

When *Not* to Self-Medicate with *Arnica*

Except for situations in which there is a clear indication for a remedy other than Arnica, there is no inappropriate time to take Arnica for a trauma.

CHAPTER TEN

Belladonna Your Homeopathic Pediatrician

"I have never been lost, but I will admit to being confused for several weeks."
—DANIEL BOONE

A good pediatrician is always there for you and your child, within reach day and night to guide you through the many concerns of childhood, from sniffles and sneezes to more serious illnesses. Like an excellent pediatrician, **Belladonna (*Atropa belladonna*)** is extremely useful for handling a broad range of childhood disorders. It provides prompt relief for problematic conditions that include fever, colds, and flu, earaches, sore throats, sunstroke, heat prostration, colic, and nightmares. Breastfeeding mothers also find it enormously helpful in relieving mastitis, or breast infection, which enables them to continue safely and comfortably nursing their infants.

When you think about *Belladonna,* remember the motto "A stitch in time saves nine." *Belladonna* states often occur in the early hours of an illness, at which time this extraordinary homeopathic remedy is capable of stopping even serious problems from progressing beyond initial fever and discomfort. A person may only need a single dose.

How can you determine that someone needs this remedy and not a comparable one, such as *Aconitum?* People requiring *Belladonna* will always demonstrate a certain level of confusion, even sedation, along with enlarged pupils and a hot, red face. As you know after reading the last chapter, this state is distinct from the one that is improved by *Aconitum.* The following description of the remedy and the plant that it is derived from will help you clearly understand the signs that indicate a need for *Belladonna.*

The Origins of *Belladonna*

Belladonna grows in both Europe and Asia. Some naturalists suggest that it originated in India. In its crude form, the plant is known and used both for its medicinal properties and hallucinogenic effects. Its Latin name, *Atropa belladonna,* is derived from two sources. *Atropa,* the genus appellation comes from the Ancient Greek word *atropos,* meaning "the inevitable." As the name of the eldest of the three Fates in Greek mythology, this is a reference to its poisonous nature. She was responsible for cutting the threads that are woven into the cloth of human life and dictating each person's ultimate destiny.

The word *belladonna* means "beautiful lady" in both Spanish and Italian. Connecting this idea with the plant probably refers to a tradition in the medieval Spanish and Italian cultures for women to dilate their pupils by placing a drop of a liquid concoction of the plant belladonna in each eye. The application made their eyes glassy, and obviously this effect was perceived as highly attractive to the men living in that historical era. The juice of the plant was also used to cause the skin to appear paler, another desired feature of women in that period.

There is another, more dangerous side of this plant's effects. Historians suggest that belladonna juice would have been a part of sleeping potions concocted in the Elizabethan era, such as the fictitious one used by the lovers in Shakespeare's play *Romeo and Juliet*. Belladonna is a member of the Solanaceae or nightshade family, which includes such menacing relatives as the hairy henbane (Hyoscyamus niger), whose raw essence is the foundation of a remedy effective in treating psychosis, and thornapple, the raw material for another useful homeopathic remedy, *Stramonium*.

Belladonna is striking in its appearance. In only a single season, its tall, hairy stem can reach a height of six feet. Leaves span up to ten inches in length. The plant flowers in July and August, producing large, bell-shaped blossoms that later turn into large shiny black berries, which reach the size of cherries by September. Due to the combination of their poisonous nature and seductive sweet taste, the berries have been called "devil's cherries" and "naughty man's cherries."

All parts of the plant are poisonous, even when taken in small quantities, and the sweet black berries are especially so. Some people have reported eating up to five of the berries and survived, but others have died from eating just one. Because the juice is so sweet it can, and has attracted the taste buds of curious children, who then fall ill. Thus, another name for belladonna is deadly nightshade, a reference at least partially derived from the number of infant deaths associated with consuming the plant's berries.

The symptoms of poisoning from the natural deadly nightshade plant have been known for centuries. These include fever, dry mouth, rapid pulse, and dilation of the pupils, headache, difficulty swallowing, hallucinations, nightmares, and convulsions, to name a few. Of course, as you understand well by now, these are exactly the kind of symptoms that homeopathically prepared *Belladonna* alleviates. "Like cures like." Based on the outcome from accidental poisonings and the results of numerous purposeful provings, today we have fully catalogued the specific picture of the *Belladonna* state.

Like other poisonous plants, belladonna is transformed into a parent's best friend as a result of the sophisticated process of serial dilutions and successions, which renders it harmless. Homeopathic preparations of *Belladonna* are completely safe—and potent. As a matter of fact, Samuel Hahnemann saved the lives of many children suffering from an epidemic of scarlet fever in 1801 using *Belladonna*. Perhaps more interestingly, he then discovered that *Belladonna* could be used to prevent future cases of the deadly illness. We'll talk more about that breakthrough discovery later, in the section on sore throats.

Symptoms Characteristic of the *Belladonna* State

Taking *Belladonna* can help any condition that begins with the following unique combination of symptoms.

- Sudden onset
- High fever
- Confusion
- Frequently sleepy, yet cannot fall asleep
- Fear of imaginary objects
- Sensitive to light, noise, and touch
- Eyes are staring, glossy with enlarged pupils

- Red, hot, dry face with cold hands and/or feet
- No thirst during high fever, otherwise thirsty for lemonade or wants lemons
- Throbbing, bursting headache
- Any inflammation with a sensation of dryness, burning heat, and bright redness

Things that make it worse are:
- Motion, even slight jarring.
- Noise.
- Light.
- Lying down.

Things that make it better are:
- Standing.
- Sitting up.

Circumstances that may trigger this combination of symptoms include:
- Any acute infection, such as a cold or flu virus.
- Exposure to sunlight and heat.

Fever

The realities of life frequently offer amazing examples of how well homeopathy works.

One evening I was walking in downtown Manhattan with a colleague, a family physician, from the Continuum Center for Health and Healing, where I worked at the time, who was "on call" for pediatrics that night. Around eight o'clock, the doctor received a page asking him to phone a couple whose child had a high fever, and he suggested that I participate. He knew basic homeopathy and wanted to be sure he did the right thing if homeopathy can be employed.

During the phone conversation, the mother told my colleague that her six-year-old daughter had been seen for a cold earlier that same day by a pediatrician at the Center. That pediatrician felt comfortable that the child didn't have a serious infection and suggested using homeopathy if a high fever developed. Now, according to the mother, the girl appeared red and hot, and had a core temperature of 102 degrees Fahrenheit. We asked her to touch her daughter's hands. They were cold. We asked about the girl's eyes. She told us that her daughter's pupils were large and her eyes looked glassy. The girl was slightly confused.

Based on the conversation we had the following information: no serious infection was found earlier that day, the fever was high, and the girl showed the signs of needing *Belladonna*. Fortunately, the woman was prepared and had a few remedies on hand. We recommended that she give the child three pellets of *Belladonna* 30C and report back to us in an hour. That report was good. The child had gone to sleep soon after receiving the dose of pellets and her fever was down. We made a suggestion to repeat the remedy using the plussing method (see Chapter 3) if the fever returned in the middle of the night. Our follow-up call the next day revealed no problems. The child was well.

Guess what? You could have done as good a job as we did and perhaps would face an even easier decision. After all, you have an advantage: You can see your little patient right in front of you. You also have the same safeguard if the problem continues: your pediatrician. Of course, it wouldn't hurt if your pediatrician read this book, too.

Belladonna is the homeopathic remedy most frequently needed to treat fever in children. Like *Aconitum*, it is most beneficial in the first twenty-four to forty-eight hours of fever. But its picture can be easily distinguished from the *Aconitum* picture. Someone who needs *Belladonna* has glassy eyes with enlarged pupils (compare this symptom to small pupils in the case of *Aconitum*). Those who need *Aconitum* are morbidly scared and extremely restless.

Symptoms are usually clear and include some degree of confusion, high fever, and feeling and looking hot and dry. Some people may hallucinate and even become angry and bite. In some cases, you may notice slight twitching of the face and the body, or even febrile seizures. There is no thirst at the height of the fever. But at other times people frequently ask for lemonade or lemons.

Let's briefly consider five other frequently indicated and easy-to-distinguish remedies.

Aconitum napellus **(monkshood):** Symptoms frequently begin after exposure to a chilling wind. In this state, the person is excited, afraid, and restless. If this individual isn't excited and restless, *Aconitum* probably isn't a good choice of remedy.

Characteristic symptoms are:
- Sudden onset.
- Fear, especially fear of death (usually for no reason).
- Restlessness.
- Small pupils.
- Chill or extremely high fever.
- Tremendous thirst.

Table 10.1 Fever Remedy Comparison Chart

Remedy	Onset	Better	Worse
Aconitum	Sudden	Open air	Exposure to cold air; warm room; evening/night, after midnight
Belladonna	Sudden	Lemonade; lemons	Afternoon, especially around 3 PM
Bryonia	Slow progression	Being alone (emotionally better)	Slightest movement; 9 PM
Chamomilla	Sudden	Being carried (emotionally better)	Dentition; being uncovered
Ferrum phosphoricum	Frequently sudden	Characteristically, no modalities	Characteristically, no modalities

***Bryonia alba* (white bryony):** Used for slowly progressing influenza and common colds in which muscular aching is one of the important symptoms. The key indication is the desire to be absolutely still, as the patient feels much worse from even the slightest movement. The patient does everything possible to save energy.

Emotional State	Signs Guiding Your Selection	Reasons to Say No to This Remedy
Fearful; anxious; restless; clinging to parents from fear	Extreme fear (including fear of dying); panic; restlessness; immediately after a bite	Absence of fear and anxiety
Confused; may have hallucinations; may appear sedated	Flushed face with cold hands and feet; dilated pupils; no thirst; frequently, right-sided pounding headache	Small pupils; low-grade fever; discharges; late stages (more than 24 hours) of illness
Wants to be left alone; refuses to answer questions; irritable	Tremendous thirst; fever with the sensation of heat and profuse perspiration; chills that begin from the fingertips and toes	Communicative; no thirst
Irritable; capricious	Teething in babies and older children; intolerable heat that does not come down; diarrhea	Mild tempered; gentle; constipated
Pleasant; good natured;	With the look of *Belladonna,* but without characteristic modalities	Irritable; demanding; has unique modalities

Characteristic symptoms are:
- Feeling restless internally, but cannot tolerate even the slightest motion.
- **Wanting to be left alone,** not wanting to answer questions, being irritable without expressing it aloud.
- Fever with the pronounced sensation of heat.
- Profuse perspiration.

- Chills beginning distally (fingertips, toes, rarely the lips), and can be triggered by anger.
- Very thirsty for **large gulps** at intervals.
- Severe headaches located on the front left side of the head, or on the back of the head.
- Generally worse on the right side of the body (except for the headache, which is left-sided).
- Worse: frequently at 9 PM, and **from the slightest motion.**
- That the person is usually warm and feel worse in warm rooms.

Chamomilla **(German chamomile):** Especially useful for young children who get a fever during teething, and older kids and adults with intense, long-lasting fevers.

Characteristic symptoms in children include:
- New teeth coming in.
- Irritability and capriciousness.
- A child calms down only if carried in someone's arms.
- One cheek is red and the other pale (*only* important in combination with other characteristic symptoms—use as a final point of assessment).
- Extremely high fever with intolerable heat that does not come down for a long time.
- Face and head are hot and sweaty.
- Thirsty.
- Worse: 9 AM and/or at night, when the baby is angry, from uncovering.

Ferrum phosphoricum **(phosphate of iron):** The main feature of this remedy is that it has no specific symptoms other than fever. Unfortunately, this sometimes leads parents either not to use it at all or to use it every time their child has a fever. What's the real deal? A few hours after your child gets a fever, if you cannot find anything to report more specific than "hot to touch" and "red face," odds are that your child needs *Ferrum*.

Characteristic symptoms are:
- Gradual onset of fever.
- Headache that feels better from a cold compress.
- Like those of a *Belladonna* state, but with no confusion and all the symptoms are milder.
- Worse from: motion and at night.
- Better from: cold applications and lying down (compare with *Belladonna,* which is the opposite of both), and touch (Compare with *Bryonia,* when a child won't let you touch them).

Sunstroke and Heat Prostration

Frequently people think that sunstroke and heat prostration are the same condition. Actually, that's not true. Sunstroke develops suddenly and severely, and includes a full, extremely rapid pulse. Heat prostration develops gradually and its presentation is less dramatic, although equally dangerous. A child left sitting inside a car could easily get heat prostration, or a child at the beach on a bright day, sunstroke. When either condition occurs, the victim must be put in the shade and cooled off as quickly as possible.

Warning: If someone's skin is dry and very hot, or if the body temperature is rising super rapidly, the situation can become life threatening. First aid is to pour cool water on the victim, apply ice, and give ice-cold drinks. Calling 911 is a must. Then, while waiting for help to arrive, give the sufferer a homeopathic remedy.

Belladonna is indicated when there are high fever, burning dry and flushed skin, enlarged pupils, and a strong and rapid pulse. Frequently *Belladonna*-type sunstroke develops after a person falls asleep in the sun. The sufferer might also exhibit confusion and all the other typical signs of *Belladonna*, including a pulsating headache. If someone in this condition becomes agitated (rare), *Belladonna* is almost a 100 percent correct choice.

Here are six of the most helpful alternative choices.

***Aconitum napellus* (monkshood):** If you see symptoms of tremendous fear of death in combination with agitation (a rare occurrence in sunstroke victims), *Aconitum* would be your first choice. In this case:
- Sunstroke comes on suddenly and with a violent intensity.
- Pupils are constricted.

***Carbo vegetabilis* (vegetable charcoal):** *Carbo* is appropriate if:
- There are fainting and collapse—under any circumstances.
- A heat or sunstroke victim becomes cold, clammy, and nauseous.
- An individual is much better from fanning.

***Cuprum metallicum* (copper):** Consider *Cuprum* if symptoms include:
- Severe cramps in the abdomen and/or legs.
- Face is pale.
- Extreme weakness. (Compare to *Veratrum*.)

***Gelsemium sempervirens* (yellow jasmine):** For the profile of a *Gelsemium* the most characteristic symptom is a headache in the back of the head. There is also likely to be:
- Severe weakness.

- Feeling of trembling.
- Vertigo and dizziness.

Glonoine **(nitroglycerine):** The primary remedy for sunstroke. A *Glonoine* state typically includes:
- Violent pulsating headache with a feeling that the head will burst any time.
- Similar symptoms to a *Belladonna* state, but the headache is significantly more violent.
- Headache that feels better when wearing a hat.
- Hotness and drowsiness.
- Frequent desire for urination.

Veratrum album **(white hellebore):** Most useful in cases of heat exhaustion, which usually results from dehydration. The pulse is not as pounding as in sunstroke (it doesn't go higher than one hundred beats per minute), and:
- The skin is cold and clammy.
- The victim is pale, weak, and nauseous.

Earache

Earache usually signals the inflammation of the middle ear, or *otitis media*. Although this condition is often called *acute* otitis media (AOM), logically only the first episode can be considered acute. All subsequent cases in the same individual most probably indicate the development of a chronic condition. Prompt homeopathic treatment of the first episode usually halts the development of chronic earaches. If more than one earache does occur, it is imperative to see a trained homeopath to cure the chronic otitis. Untreated infections in the ears are potentially dangerous, as they can develop into meningitis, an inflammation of the membranes covering the brain and the spinal cord.

Pediatricians increasingly embrace the tactic of watchful waiting. If a child doesn't show obvious signs of severe infection, the pediatrician refrains from prescribing an antibiotic right away. This window of opportunity is a good time to try a homeopathic solution. You should also remember that the first symptoms, which only you get to see, could respond to homeopathy and quickly eliminate the ground for any future issues.

Belladonna is the main homeopathic remedy for the sudden onset of a **right-sided earache**. In this state, someone has a high fever, a flushed face, and glassy eyes with enlarged pupils. The patient's lips are dry. Although the pain of the earache has a throbbing quality, very young children won't be able to appreciate or describe this distinction. So look closely at their behavior. Small children just grab onto or rub their right ears. Your child may be confused, have nightmares, and feel angry. In this state children often wake up screaming from fear and pain. Loud noises, touch, and light make it feel worse. It feels better when lying down (compare symptoms to *Chamomilla*).

Here are a few other important remedies for treatment of earaches.

Aconitum napellus **(monkshood):** Indicated for a sudden onset of severe pain after exposure to cold wind or draft. Also look for:
- Sudden onset.
- The child is scared, restless.
- High fever.
- Severe pain.
- Flushed face.
- Small pupils.
- Significant thirst for cold drinks.

Chamomilla **(German chamomile):** Often indicated for earaches that accompany teething. Characteristically the child who needs *Chamomilla* is:
- Highly irritable, demanding, and capricious (in other words, the child asks for something, but refuses it the moment it is offered).
- Screaming violently and calms down only if carried.
- Unwilling to be touched or even looked at.
- Worse: from lying down.

Ferrum phosphoricum **(phosphate of iron):** One of the most useful remedies at the beginning of an earache when you clearly see that there's a problem but it doesn't match any remedy you know. Although the picture of the condition is similar to the *Belladonna* state, it doesn't fit exactly—especially in the level of intensity. It just doesn't present the clear picture that someone who needs *Belladonna* usually does.

Pain is usually on the right side.

Hepar sulphuris calcareum **(calcium sulphate):** With the *Hepar* state, a child:
- Is extremely sensitive to the slightest interference. A cold draft, uncovering a part of a body, or a touch can make the pain a hundred times worse.
- Quickly flies into a rage (compare to *Chamomilla*. The child who needs *Chamomilla* calms down if constantly carried around. The *Hepar* child just doesn't want to be touched or bothered in any way. Carrying such a child will only make things worse).

Table 10.2 Earache Remedy Comparison Chart

Remedy	Onset	Better	Worse
Aconitum	Sudden	No specific modalities	No specific modalities
Belladonna	Sudden	Warm applications	Jarring; after midnight
Chamomilla	Sudden	Being carried (emotionally better)	Dentition; being uncovered
Ferrum phosphoricum	Frequently sudden	Characteristically, no modalities	Characteristically, no modalities
Hepar sulphuris	Sudden	Ear and the rest of the body being wrapped to protect from the slightest motion of the air; warmth	Movement of cold air around the ear; night

Emotional State	Signs Guiding Your Selection	Reasons to Say No to This Remedy
Scared; restless	Symptoms appear more often on left side; sudden onset with severe pain, high fever, flushed face, small pupils; afraid; significant thirst for cold drinks	Gradual onset; enlarged pupils
Confused (could even be hallucinating)	Symptoms appear more often on right side; high fever; severe pulsating pain; often, red ear; red, hot face with cold extremities; glassy eyes with large pupils; no thirst	Small pupils; low-grade fever; discharges; late stages (more than 24 hours) of illness
Very angry and demanding (this little tyrant torments the family)	Extreme sensitivity to pain; violent screaming from pain; irritability; demandingness; capriciousness	Mild mannered child
Usually sweet disposition but no specific symptoms	Symptoms most often appear on right side; sudden onset with high fever; may appear to need *Belladonna* but no modalities	Clear modalities indicating other remedies
Irritable; extremely sensitive to pain (screams from pain)	Extreme sensitivity to even the slightest motion of the air and to cold; pain made better by nothing except for being covered; desire to have the ear bundled up; sensation of a splinter stuck in ear	Desire to be uncovered; better from being carried

Table 10.2 Earache Remedy Comparison Chart *(continued)*

Pulsatilla	Gradual	Open or cool air; being gently held and gently carried	Heat; night
Verbascum	Nonspecific	No specific modalities	Biting hard; sneezing; talking

***Pulsatilla nigricans* (wind flower):** The most frequently required remedy in cases of earache that arise after the child has a "cold" with yellowish-greenish nasal discharge. With *Pulsatilla*, the child:
- Is weepy and needs affection.
- Is sweet and looks defenseless.
- Worse: from heat (compare to *Magnesia phosphorica*).
- Better: from fresh air and being gently carried (compare to the *Chamomilla* state. Here a child would have been carried in a brisk, energetic way).

***Verbascum thapsus* (mullein):** Indicative of a *Verbascum* state is:
- Left-sided earache.
- Hoarseness, and possibly a deep-toned cough.
- Worsening from sitting, change of temperature, talking, biting teeth together, and in the evening.
- Better after rising from a sitting position and from taking a deep breath.

Mild mannered; weepy; wants affection and consolation	More common in left ear; ear infection that begins with cold and greenish discharge from the nose; weepiness; mild mannered; need for attention	Anger; desire not to be touched; likes heat
No specific picture	Severe left-sided earache; hoarse voice; deep-toned cough	Right-sided complaints

Sore Throat

Belladonna is an absolute leader in the treatment of acute sore throats. As I mentioned at the start of the chapter, Hahnemann became a veritable medical celebrity in 1801 due to his discovery of the tremendous value of homeopathic *Belladonna* in treating scarlet fever, a severe form of strep throat. Only five years after homeopathy's official inception, an epidemic swept Germany. Children were the main victims. Through an experience in caring for children within the same family, some who got ill and some who did not, he identified the curative power of *Belladonna* for most of the cases of scarlet fever occurring at that time.

Hahnemann achieved such impressive results in the treatment and prevention of deadly scarlet fever in 1801, in fact, that many allopathic physicians soon adopted his new approach and began praising homeopathy. The outcome was staggering. Ten physicians gave homeopathic *Belladonna* to 1,646 children for preventative care, and they reported that only 123 patients developed the illness. Whereas the morbidity rate in the untreated population surged as high as 90 percent!

Subsequently, the top public health official in Germany declared the remedy effective. Other doctors were encouraged to adopt it.

Please don't rush out and start dosing your children willy-nilly with *Belladonna* this winter in hopes of avoiding strep throat. Later on Hahnemann and other homeopaths realized that the *Belladonna* success was merely a temporary solution. In many cases of strep throat other remedies are required. It depends on the individual characteristics of the patient and the particular epidemiological situation in a particular area.

Bear in mind that homeopaths do not prescribe remedies for specific conditions, but rather for individual patients. It is only in rare cases of epidemics, when there are so many people at once suffering from an illness that a common remedy picture emerges. However, the remedy is a specific only during that particular epidemic. Even if both are having outbreaks of the same disease, *Belladonna* might be the right match for a New Jersey community while another remedy might be right for a community in Kansas.

Typical symptoms that call for the use of *Belladonna* for the treatment of a sore throat include:

- Pain and burning on the right side.
- Intolerance for even a slight touch of the throat.
- High fever with a red face.
- Large pupils.
- Hot red head, and cold hands and feet.
- Confusion.

Seven other helpful remedies for the same types of conditions are:

***Aconitum napellus* (monkshood):** Look at *Aconitum* when:
- The sore throat begins suddenly after exposure to cold, windy weather.

- The symptoms are very severe.
- The child is scared and restless
- The child is thirsty for cold drinks that are painful to swallow (compare with *Phytolacca decandra*).

Ferrum phosphoricum (phosphate of iron): The most specific symptom of this remedy is a lack of specific symptoms. Use for:
- Sore throat with high to moderate fever.
- Gradual onset of the illness.
- Significant weakness.
- No specific symptoms that point to any other remedy you know.

Hepar sulphuris calcareum (calcium sulfate): *Hepar* is indicated for symptoms of:
- Extreme irritability at the slightest provocation, and extreme sensitivity to pain and suffering.
- Feeling chilly, with cold sweat.
- Splinter-like pains in the throat. A child might say: "I have a fish-bone in my throat." (Of course, make sure this isn't true, because if it is, then the remedy isn't what is needed; rather the bone has to be removed.)
- Liquids feel OK to swallow, solids cause pain. (Compare with *Lachesis muta*.)

Lachesis muta (bushmaster snake venom): A great remedy discovered by Dr. Hering. Use for:
- Exclusively left-sided symptoms.
- Neck is very sensitive. Cannot tolerate even a slight pressure from tight collars.
- Worse from swallowing saliva and hot drinks, on waking up, and heat.
- Better from cold drinks and temporary relief from swallowing solid food. (Compare with *Hepar sulphuris*.)

Table 10.3 Sore Throat Remedy Comparison Chart

Remedy	Onset	Better	Worse
Aconitum	Sudden	No specific modalities	Cold drinks that are highly desired but painful to swallow
Belladonna	Sudden	No specific modalities	Touch to the throat; any motion that involves the throat area; swallowing liquids
Ferrum phosphoricum	Sudden	No specific modalities	Night
Hepar sulphuris	Sudden	Warm drinks; warm wraps of the throat	Cold drinks; movement of cold air around throat; night
Lachesis	At night or on waking up	Cold drinks; very brief relief from swallowing	Waking up; touching the throat; tight collars; night (may wake up in the middle of the night from being sick)

Emotional State	Signs Guiding Your Selection	Reasons to Say No to This Remedy
Scared; restless	Sudden onset; high fever; flushed face; small pupils; feeling of terror; significant thirst for cold drinks	Gradual onset; enlarged pupils
Confused (could even be hallucinating)	Sudden onset of right-sided complaints; red, hot face with cold extremities; large pupils; no thirst	Thirst; small pupils
Usually sweet disposition; no specific symptoms	Significant weakness; prostration	Clear modalities indicating other remedies
Irritable	Extreme sensitivity to even the slightest motion of the air and cold; desire to stay bundled up with the throat covered; sensation of constriction of a splinter in the throat	Desire to be uncovered; better from cold drinks (think about *Phytolacca* or *Lachesis*)
Intense; can be very talkative (can't stop talking despite the pain)	Exclusively for left-sided pain or when the problem starts on the left and goes to the right; sensation of constriction of a lump in the throat; lump in the throat; possibly, purple-covered tonsils	Relaxed feeling; right-sided complaints; no feeling of constriction

Table 10.3 Sore Throat Remedy Comparison Chart *(continued)*

Remedy	Onset	Better	Worse
Mercurius vivus (often for right-sided pain)	No specific timing	No specific modalities	Swallowing; heat; warmth of bed; extreme warmth or cold; night
Mercurius iodatus ruber (exclusively for left-sided pain)	No specific timing	No specific modalities	Same as *Mercurius vivus*
Phytolacca (often for right-sided pain)	No specific timing	Cold drinks	Hot drinks

Mercurius vivus **(quicksilver):** Indicated for:
- Right-sided sore throats most frequently (but not always).
- Slow onset.
- Offensive breath.
- Increased salivation, especially at night.
- Increased perspiration.
- Dirty looking, thick, coated tongue with teeth imprints on the edges.
- Metallic taste.
- Neck glands are frequently swollen and tender.
- Much worse at night and with empty swallowing.

Emotional State	Signs Guiding Your Selection	Reasons to Say No to This Remedy
No specific modalities related to acute illness	Offensive breath; intense drooling, especially at night; swollen, painful glands on the neck; metallic taste; coated, dirty-looking tongue with tooth imprints; significant perspiration	Lack of specific symptoms
No specific modalities	Similar to *Mercurius vivus*	Right-sided tonsillitis without typical mercurial symptoms
No specific modalities	Burning, raw throat; enlarged glands on the neck	Can drink hot liquids; no feeling of burning in the throat

***Mercurius iodatus ruber* (biniodide of mercury):** Points of consideration are:
- Frequently indicated for left-sided sore throat.
- All other symptoms are similar to *Mercurius vivus*.

***Phytolacca decandra* (poke root):** Use when:
- Throat is raw, swollen, and burning.
- Painful swallowing that radiates into ears.
- Feeling of the hot lump.
- Pain at the root of the tongue and/or on the palate right above the tongue.
- Tongue is coated with the red tip.
- Worse: from hot drinks.

- Better: from cold drinks.
- The glands on the neck are frequently enlarged and painful (similar to both of the *Mercurius* remedies).

A Few More Conditions That May Require *Belladonna*

An amazingly large number of babies with colic require the administration of *Belladonna*. The key symptom to look for is that they get better from lying on the belly. You can read more about this ailment in Chapter 11, "Chamomilla."

Another serious problem that a large number of children in the modern world face is nightmares. Although not described in great detail in this book, this problem frequently responds to a single dose of *Belladonna*, provided that the child presents with other characteristic symptoms of this remedy. Bear in mind, however, that another important remedy to consider for nightmares is *Stramonium*. Almost for certain, the combination of terrible nightmares, night terrors, fear of the dark, and fear of dogs indicates a need for *Stramonium*.

Belladonna can be helpful with a large number of acute and chronic ailments ranging from seizure disorders to ovarian cysts and sinusitis, but finding a correct remedy for these conditions should be left up to a professional homeopath.

When *Not* to Self-Medicate with *Belladonna*

Do not give *Belladonna* to yourself or anyone else when:
- The person is weak, and the reaction to the illness is also weak with gradual onset of symptoms.
- There is no high fever and there are no changes in the mental-emotional sphere.
- Faced with a chronic condition, or a complex set of conditions.

CHAPTER ELEVEN

Chamomilla Your Homeopathic Babysitter

"I am sorry to say that Peter was not very well during the evening. His mother put him to bed, and made some chamomile tea; and she gave a dose of it to Peter! 'One tablespoon to be taken at bedtime.'"
—BEATRIX POTTER, *THE TALE OF PETER RABBIT*

Chamomilla (*Matricaria recutita*, German chamomile) has been known for centuries for its calming effect on children. That's why we're calling it a homeopathic babysitter—and a good one, too. Chamomilla can help your child get through colic and problems with teething. It relieves pain, subdues anger, and eases the fear of a child frightened of dentists and surgeons. The children (and sometimes the adults) who need *Chamomilla* always act enormously irritable, angry, demanding, and capricious.

You can easily recognize a child who needs *Chamomilla* just from hearing shocking screams in the background while you're having a phone conversation with a friend who has a baby or a toddler. In adults, another good example of the *Chamomilla* state would be the pregnant woman who screams her lungs out during childbirth, cursing at her husband and everyone else in the delivery room for "all the pain they've caused." A woman in this state asks for something she "really needs" and then rejects it the moment it's been brought to her. She's impulsive, unpredictable, and inconsistent.

The Origins of *Chamomilla*

Native to Europe and Asia, German chamomile has been grown successfully in Australia and North America. Some gardeners call it *true chamomile,* as it frequently is confused with so-called Roman chamomile, a plant many people use for making lawns, because the more you run on it the faster it grows. But German and Roman chamomile actually belong to different species. Egyptians worshiped chamomile for its medicinal properties, which were rediscovered by Europeans in the Middle Ages when it was applied to children's ailments, nausea, nervous complaints, and skin diseases. In that period, it was also considered to be helpful for diseases of the kidneys and spleen, bladder troubles, colds, malaria, and to expel worms. Chamomile tea was believed to make an excellent wash for sore and weak eyes. It was also used as a poultice for pain and swellings.[1]

In *The New Honest Herbal,* Varro E. Tyler writes about herbal chamomile: "As a popular remedy, it may be thought of as the European counterpart of ginseng."[2] He also mentions that the Germans call the plant *alles zutraut,* "everything is possible." Traditionally chamomile root was chewed to reduce toothache.

Gardeners who practice the biodynamic method of growing plants use German chamomile as an important fertilizer. Drooping and dying plants have been observed to recover if German chamomile is planted near them. It also stimulates the growth of grain. Old herbal books called chamomile the "plant physician."

Unlike aconitum and belladonna, the German chamomile plant does not have an impressive, dangerous, or distinguished look, rather it looks like the kind of wild flower whose petals a lover plucks when pining, "She loves me, she loves me not." It is a strange contradiction that a beautiful plant would be so useful for patients who are a disaster. We expect pregnant women or an innocent child to be angelic, and our expectations are defied when they behave like devils. Heaven meets hell. Considering the long history of the allopathic use of this herb to soothe severe complaints and its innocent look, you would probably not expect it to cause severe symptoms, exactly opposite from its appearance.

Symptoms Characteristic of the *Chamomilla* State

Eminent American homeopath Margaret Tyler wrote: "An excellent name for Chamomilla is 'cannot bear it' —Can't bear himself. Can't bear other people. Can't bear pain. Can't bear things; wants them, and hurls them away. Everything is simply intolerable." She also states: "Despite this picture of gentility, this is the remedy that cannot return a civil answer."[3]

N.M. Choudhuri, a prominent Indian homeopath, called *Chamomilla* the "ugliest remedy."[4] The children—and sometimes the adults—who need homeopathic *Chamomilla* bring misery wherever they go. They have the worst temper tantrums you can possibly imagine. They scream and cry, kick and bite, throw themselves on the floor and bend backward, practically driving their parents and everyone around them to despair.

Chamomilla can help any condition that begins with the following unique combination of symptoms.

- Loud, constant screaming
- Extreme irritability
- Anger, whining, demanding
- Sensitive to even the slightest pain. Perspires from even the slightest pain. May even faint from pain.
- Does not want to be touched or spoken to
- Capricious (asks for things that are immediately rejected when delivered)
- Worse from sun, open air, **night**, heat
- Better from being constantly carried. Toothache is better from cold.

You may have heard or read about an unusual characteristic of the *Chamomilla* state: one cheek hot and red, the other cheek cold and pale. Although this symptom is described in every single book I've read on homeopathy, people rarely develop it. I have never seen this symptom in my twenty-plus years of private practice. Some people do develop it, just not often. Of course, if you ever do see this particular indicator in combination with other important traits of the Chamomilla state, you can use it to confirm your choice. However, if you see all the other symptoms except for this one please go ahead and give the remedy. You likely still have a match.

Circumstances that involve this combination of symptoms may include:

- Teething.
- Earache.
- Colic.
- Childbirth: when a woman is screaming and yelling from severe, intolerable pain, look for other key symptoms of Chamomilla.
- Diarrhea (also see Chapter 14, "Nux Vomica").

Screaming Babies

We all know too well how disturbing a screaming baby can be. Babies cannot tell us what is wrong. We know they are suffering, but it is hard to understand the reason. My first wife and I had a baby like this and, I'll tell you, we had to come up with various sophisticated ways to calm her down. If you have a screaming baby, please ensure that there's nothing seriously wrong going on. A visit to a pediatrician is an excellent idea, as a first step.

The overwhelming majority of screaming babies come out of the pediatrician's office the same way they went in: screaming and with parents and a doctor who have no clue about what's going on. But they do have an important piece of information! There is nothing terribly wrong or else the pediatrician would detect it. They also know the baby is in pain. But they don't know why. In newborns, extended screaming is called colic. In older infants this behavior is usually due to teething. Both conditions may be accompanied by diarrhea or constipation.

Homeopathy can do miracles for screaming babies. The key to selecting a remedy in such cases is to try to understand what makes the baby feel better or feel worse. If you have tried your best without a result, it is a good time to visit a professional homeopath.

A screaming baby in a *Chamomilla* state shows characteristics typical of the remedy. Most of the babies are healthy and react to the reason that causes pain in a distinct manner. I will always remember the screams of a baby who needs *Chamomilla*. The sound is loud and demanding. It can only be stopped by holding or rocking the baby, and walking around. The moment you put the baby down the screaming begins again.

Frequently babies in this state indicate—and toddlers tell you—that they want something, but immediately reject it if you bring it in. You simply cannot please this group. They are sensitive to noise and odors. They start to nurse, then become irritable and pull off. They may bite the nipple or strike you if they are older. Teething and colic in combination with green, spinach-like diarrhea, or teething with earache are common signs that your baby or toddler would benefit from taking *Chamomilla*.

When dosing an infant remember to try the plussing method described in Chapter 3, where the remedy is diluted in water. Another, more "material" way to administer homeopathy to babies than that is to crush three pellets of a concentration 30C remedy between two spoons, add a drop of water, and spoon feed the mixture to the child.

One dose of Chamomilla 30C is usually sufficient to soothe a screaming infant. If you see an improvement and then the baby complains again (screams) in a few hours or the next day, repeat the dose. With the correct remedy the need for repetition will become less and less frequent. Often one dose of the remedy takes care of the entire problem.

Now let's talk about other options for screaming babies who do not present with a typical *Chamomilla* picture.

Colic

Amy Rothenberg, N.D., a respected homeopath and naturopathic physician who treats a lot of children, frequently asks the mothers of colicky babies to drink some nonalcoholic beer a half-hour or so before nursing.[5] In her experience this helps the mother to relax due, most probably, to the ingredient hops. I suggest drinking hops tea instead of beer. The main objective here is to break the cycle of a nervous mother, which leads to a crying baby, which in turn leads to a nervous mother and crying baby, and so on.

Sometimes a baby will do better if the nursing mother avoids vegetables in the *Brassicaceae* family: horseradish, radish, pak-choi (Chinese mustard), pe tsai (Chinese cabbage), spinach mustard, turnip, broccoli, kale, cauliflower, cabbage, Brussels sprouts, kohlrabi, watercress. Although not members of the same family, onions and garlic are not recommended either. If the baby is on a formula, changing it can help.

Many of you already know about such precautions: remove certain foods from the diet, change the baby formula . . . but your baby still has colic! What can you do? Now is the time to turn to homeopathy.

As you proceed, remember that seeing the lack of a complete improvement after homeopathy may be not the result of giving your child the wrong remedy—although that is possible. Instead it could be due to a birth trauma to the head and spine, or dietary intolerances, such as allergies to milk, soy, or something in the mom's diet.

We already discussed necessary dietary adjustments for mother and child. If you suspect birth trauma, a visit to a good osteopath who does cranial-sacral therapy may also bring about a dramatic improvement.

Here are eleven homeopathic remedies that could also apply if *Chamomilla* is not the answer.

Aethusa cynapium **(fool's parsley):** Often the right remedy for babies who are unable to tolerate milk or mother's milk. Indications to use this remedy include:

- **Vomits milk in curds soon after nursing.**
- Gets colicky and irritable after vomiting and then may go too sleep.
- Hungry after vomiting.
- Vomiting may be accompanied by greenish diarrhea.

- Worse: evening and 3 AM to 4 AM, from exertion and hot weather.

Belladonna **(deadly nightshade):** If necessary, review Chapter 9. Indications to use this remedy include:
- **Distended, hot abdomen with protruding lumps.**
- Face is hot, red and dry.
- Dilated pupils.
- Sensitive to jarring, light, noise. (Compare to Chamomilla, who wants to be rocked.)
- May have high fever.
- Violent pains come in waves: appear and disappear suddenly.
- Worse: from touch, pressure, lying on belly.
- Better: from bending backward, dark room, rest.

Bryonia alba **(white bryony):** This presentation may remind you a lot of *Chamomilla*. The main differences between the remedies are:
- Slightest motion (even coughing) creates severe pain.
- Wants to be left alone (compare to *Chamomilla* and *Pulsatilla nigricans*).
- Very thirsty. (Compare to *Pulsatilla nigricans.*)

Cina **(wormseed):** May remind you of *Chamomilla* in its presentation. The main differences are:
- Hard abdomen.
- Dissatisfied, angry, does not want to be looked at.
- **Always hungry,** but develops diarrhea or vomiting after food.
- Grinding of teeth or gums.
- Itching anus and/or nose.
- Better from lying on the abdomen, motion, being carried (compare to Chamomilla).

- Worse from touch, **much worse at night. Frequently the babies are OK all day, but they scream their lungs out at night.**

Colocynthis **(bitter cucumber):** Indications to use it include:
- Writhing in pain, pulls legs up to the abdomen.
- Extremely irritable, restless, but does not calm down if carried (compare to Chamomilla and Pulsatilla nigricans).
- Colic after anger.
- Better: **from hard pressure** (parents hoist the baby up and over the shoulder to provide hard pressure), bending forward.
- Worse: at night, lying on the abdomen.

Ignatia amara **(St. Ignatius' bean):** For a colicky baby whose mother has endured a significant loss (for example, a divorce or the death of her husband, mother, close relative, or friend) during pregnancy or breastfeeding. Another common stressful situation is immigration or a relocation during which personal connections are severed and the mother grieves the loss of friends. A dose of Ignatia amara 30C for the baby and 200C for the mother may relieve the colic and ease the mother's emotional pain.

Table 11.1 Colic Remedy Comparison Chart

Remedy	Onset	Better	Worse
Aethusa	Soon after feeding	Company; open air	Heat; summer; evening
Belladonna	Comes and goes suddenly	Lying on the belly; bending (forward or backward)	Jarring
Bryonia	No particular pattern	Lying still	Slightest motion (even a parent trying to sit on the bed)
Chamomilla (the most common remedy)	Sudden	Being constantly carried and rocked	Being left alone; night
Cina	Sudden	Lying on the belly; being carried over the shoulder; daytime	Night

Emotional State	Signs Guiding Your Selection	Remedy to Compare with
Irritable; crying	Vomits curds of milk soon after nursing; gets colicky, irritable, exhausted, and then goes to sleep	*Pulsatilla*
Confused (could even be hallucinating)	Pains that appear/disappear suddenly; improvement from lying on the belly; distending abdomen with protruding lumps	*Cina*
Irritable; wants to be left alone	Much worse from even the slightest motion; thirst for cold drinks	*Chamomilla*
Restless; very angry and demanding (this little tyrant torments the family)	Extreme sensitivity to pain; angry crying with arching of the back; desire to be constantly carried and rocked	*Cina*; *Colocynthis*; *Rheum*
Angry; does not want to be looked at	OK all day and then scream lungs out all night; always hungry	*Belladonna*; *Chamomilla*, *Rheum*, *Jalapa* (a rare remedy characterized by baby who seems to sleep all day and cry all night)

Table 11.1 Colic Remedy Comparison Chart *(continued)*

Remedy	Onset	Better	Worse
Colocynthis (a common remedy)	Sudden	Hard pressure; bending forward; thrashing about; heat	Night
Ignatia	No specific timing	Eating (paradoxical modality)	Warm application; morning
Lycopodium	4 to 8 PM	Warm applications; warm drinks; passing gas and/or burping (which provide temporary relief)	Eating
Nux vomica	Morning	Bowel movement; warm applications	Before passing a stool
Magnesium phosphoricum (a common remedy)	Sudden	Warm, even hot, applications; bending double; hard pressure	Cold; touch; night
Pulsatilla	Gradual	Being gently held and gently carried; nursing	Heat; night

Emotional State	Signs Guiding Your Selection	Reasons to Say No to This Remedy
Irritable; extremely restless from pain	Severe pain (pulls legs up to the abdomen and thrashes about in pain); not better from being carried; better from hard pressure	*Belladonna; Cina; Chamomilla; Magnesium*
Changeable emotional state	Babies of mothers who are under significant emotional stress or in a family where there is a lot of stress (arguments, divorce, death)	*Chamomilla*
Looks anxious with wrinkled brow	Abdominal distention with gurgling and gas	*Pulsatilla*
Irritable; very sensitive to all external stimuli impressions	Colic before stool or when attempting to pass a stool	*Chamomilla; Colocynthis; Rheum*
Significantly milder than those who need *Colocynthis*	Much improvement from warm applications on the abdomen	*Colocynthis*
Gentle; tearful; seeks comfort from mother	Mild mannered; much improvement from being carried gently and from nursing	*Chamomilla*

Table 11.1 Colic Remedy Comparison Chart *(continued)*

Remedy	Onset	Better	Worse
Rheum	Sudden	Bending double; warmth	Uncovering; eating; moving

Lycopodium **(club moss):** Indications to use this remedy include:
- Looking anxious, with a wrinkled brow and a worried expression.
- Bloating.
- Better from passing gas or burping, from warm bottle held to the belly.
- Worse from 4 PM to 8 PM, 2 AM, or sometimes all night.

Nux vomica **(Quaker's button):** Indications to use this remedy include:
- Constipation, has to push hard with each bowel movement.
- Anger, irritability. Carrying around or comforting does not help.
- Stuffy nose.
- Better from being very warm and drinking warm drinks.
- Worse from cold, morning, eating.

Magnesium phosphoricum (phosphate of magnesia):
- Better from warmth, warm drinks, and gentle pressure on the abdomen. This baby's colic is helped if the baby's knees can be kept up near the chest, as this seems to relieve bloating and gas. The baby will also settle down some if a good burp can be managed.

Emotional State	Signs Guiding Your Selection	Reasons to Say No to This Remedy
Dislikes one usually favorite thing, or just asks for one particular thing	Sour smell of the body and all discharges	*Chamomilla;* *Colocynthis;* *Magnesium*

- Compare with *Colocynthis,* which is better from firm pressure and doubling up.

Pulsatilla nigricans **(wind flower):** Indications to use this remedy are:
- Hiccoughs soon after eating.
- Rumbling in the belly.
- The child is much better from gentle rocking. (Compare with the *Chamomilla* state, which requires constant rocking.)
- The child is gentle, can be tearful, but does not scream, not demanding.
- Thirstless, but likes to nurse for a long time for comfort.

Rheum officinale **(rhubarb):**
- Similar to Chamomilla in changeable desires, but instead of being capricious and rejecting everything offered, the child just dislikes his or her favorite thing, or just wants one particular thing
- **The smell of the body and all the discharges (in other words, diarrhea) is sour**
- Better from bending double, warmth
- Worse from uncovering any part, eating

Teething

Some babies have absolutely no problems teething, but the majority does. For that group, homeopathic Chamomilla is the hands-down champion. Some experts believe that it is indicated in about 50 percent of cases. Nonetheless it helps only those babies who present a typical *Chamomilla* picture. Don't forget the telltale signs of *Chamomilla* children: green, spinach-like diarrhea and/or an earache that coincide with teething.

Let's look at other helpful remedies for painful and also difficult, slow teething. Remedies for slow teething should be given only once. *Dose:* Three pellets of 30C.

Aconitum napellus **(monkshood):**
- Painful teething
- High fever
- **Perspiration and thirst** (compare to *Belladonna*)
- Pupils are small
- Cheeks are hot and red, and extremities are cold
- Children toss and turn in their sleep
- Babies bite their fists, and scream

Belladonna **(deadly nightshade):**
- Painful teething
- High fever
- **No perspiration, no thirst** (compare to *Aconitum*)
- Pupils are large
- Cheeks are hot and red, and extremities are cold
- The child is angry at the pains, may bite other people and self

Calcarea carbonica **(calcium carbonate):** Indications to use this remedy include:.
- Slow, difficult teething.
- Frequent colds and coughs.
- **The child is easygoing, but stubborn.**
- Children who need this remedy are usually large or plump.
- Loves eggs, loves milk.
- Perspires on the head.

Calcarea phosphorica **(calcium phosphate):** Indications to use this remedy include:
- Slow, difficult, teething.
- Rapid tooth decay.
- Delayed closure of fontanelles on top of the head.
- **Discontent and peevish.** This child has a tendency to whine and moan. Although not correct from the purist point of view, you could call this remedy "chronic Chamomilla," as it works for more systemic, chronic cases.
- The child is usually skinny.
- Loves smoked meats, ham, and bacon.

Kreosotum **(Beachwood creosote):** The following presentation of symptoms may remind you of the Chamomilla state. The main differences are:
- Very difficult, painful teething **accompanied by coughing.**
- Cough is constant and dry.
- Fever without perspiration.
- Severe caries. Often teeth decay almost immediately after they come in.
- The child who needs *Kreosotum* is cross, willful, obstinate, and easily vexed over trifles.

Table 11.2 Teething Remedy Comparison Chart

Remedy	Onset	Better	Worse
Aconitum	Urgent	No specific modalities	No specific modalities
Belladonna	Urgent	No specific modalities	Jarring; late evening and night
Calcarea Carbonica	Chronic	Warm applications (but worse from warm food)	Warm food
Calcarea Phosporica	Chronic	Warm applications	Damp, cold weather
Chamomilla (the most common remedy)	Urgent	Being constantly carried and rocked; cold drinks	At night in bed; cold air; warm food and drinks; night
Kreosotum	Urgent	Warm applications; motion	Cold; rest

SUPER REMEDIES

Emotional State	Signs Guiding Your Selection	Reasons to Say No to This Remedy
Screams; bites own fists	High fever; small pupils; perspiration and thirst; interestingly, tooth pain in nursing mothers	*Belladonna; Chamomilla*
Angry when in pain; might try to bite other people	High fever; large pupils; no perspiration; no thirst	*Aconitum; Chamomilla Phytolacca*
Easygoing but very stubborn	Slow, painful dentition in a large child who is easygoing and loves eggs and milk; perspiration on the head; stubbornness	*Calcarea phosphorica; Silica*
Discontented and peevish	Slow painful dentition in a skinny, whining, moaning child who loves smoked meats, ham, and bacon; perspiration on the head	*Calcarea carbonica; Chamomilla* (many call *Calcarea phosphorica* remedy chronic Chamomilla); *Silica*
Irritable; screaming; wants to be carried all the time; capricious	Extreme sensitivity to pain; angry crying with arching of teh back; need to be constantly carried and rocked; dentition that is frequently accompanied by colic with green diarrhea	*Belladonna; Calcarea phosphorica*
Cross; willful; asks for many things, but throws them all away (capricious)	Painful dentition accompanied by coughing; teeth that decay very quickly	*Chamomilla*

Table 11.2 Teething Remedy Comparison Chart *(continued)*

Remedy	Onset	Better	Worse
Phytolacca	Urgent	Biting something	No specific modalities for this condition
Rheum	Urgent	Being constantly carried	At night in bed
Silica	Chronic	Warm applications	Warm drinks; biting

Phytolacca decandra (poke root): This is a remedy for acute teething problems. Its main indication is an irresistible urge to bite the teeth (or gums) together, and sometimes also to bite people, but without typical *Belladonna* symptoms. The motivation is just to bite, not to hurt anyone.

Rheum officinale (rhubarb): Although the picture is similar to *Chamomilla,* major distinctions include:
- Painful teething with colic and sour pasty diarrhea.
- The child and all the discharges have a sour smell.
- Child's mood is also pretty "sour."

Emotional State	Signs Guiding Your Selection	Reasons to Say No to This Remedy
No specific modalities for this condition	Need to bite something (frequently winds up biting own teeth or gums, or other people, but not from anger like *Belladonna*)	*Belladonna*
Irritable, "sour" mood; specifically dislikes things that were once preferred or specifically asks for a particular thing	Sour smell of the body and all discharges; combination of teething with colic and sour, pasty diarrhea	*Chamomilla*
Irritable and stubborn; can be very shy	Frequent infections; disproportionately large head in a skinny, sickly child; offensive perspiration, especially of feet	*Calcarea carbonica; Calcarea phosphorica*

Silica **(silicon dioxide):** Indications to use this remedy include:
- Slow, difficult teething.
- Frequent colds and coughs (compare to *Calcarea carbonica*).
- The child is bright, but shy and stubborn.
- Perspires on head and neck.
- **Feet frequently perspire profusely and give off an unpleasant smell.**
- Clammy hands.
- Feeling chilled.

A Few More Conditions That May Require *Chamomilla*

While most people, using conventional logic, might presume that the best homeopathic remedy to reverse the negative effects of caffeine, such as the jitters and insomnia, would be the preparation *Coffea cruda,* in reality *Chamomilla* is the best antidote. This proves that homeopathy employs the principles of "similars," not the principle of "the same."

I don't know about you, but I am afraid of dentists. They drill, you know, and that can be painful. As a child I couldn't tolerate dental pain and drilling at all. Unfortunately, my parents and doctors knew nothing about homeopathy. Well, you and I know what to do, don't we? Here is an interesting case that was aided by *Chamomilla.*

Four-year-old Alex had been a patient of mine for a while. In that time, he'd made tremendous progress from being a sickly boy with serious sinusitis and asthma to being a much stronger young gentleman. At the time of this episode, my communication with his mother was mostly on the phone about twice a year. Whenever Alex got a cold of some kind, she'd call to ask what to do. Acute homeopathic prescribing always did the trick.

On this occasion, Alex was scheduled to see a dentist the next morning, but had suddenly developed a severe earache. His mom called my cell phone at 10 PM for help. Fortunately for her and Alex, but unfortunately for my ears, I easily picked up a terrible sound. Alex was screaming like a whale! If I hadn't known this woman and the principles of homeopathy, I might have called 911 to report an attempted murder. I suggested that Alex's mother move away from the little screamer so I could hear the full story.

Well, Alex was in pain. He was rubbing his ear, had a high fever, and was experiencing diarrhea that looked like a green, kind of unformed stool. You guessed it already, I'm sure. These are characteristics of *Chamomilla*. I decided to make certain and asked what was making Alex feel better. His mom told me that giving him his favorite toys was useless, he threw them away one by one as they arrived. The only thing that worked was constantly carrying him around or rocking him. That clinched it.

I prescribed a dose of *Chamomilla* 30C for Alex to be repeated in fifteen minutes if his improvement was less than 50 percent. It worked. Alex got better quickly and we were all able to go to sleep afterwards. The next day, in the morning, his mom gave Alex one more dose of *Chamomilla*. It worked beautifully. They went to see the dentist and the boy behaved like an angel. The dentist was impressed.

Listen. I don't want anybody else to call me at night with a baby screaming bloody murder in the background. Please learn about *Chamomilla!* OK?

With the advances of modern dentistry, toothaches are becoming much rarer. Nonetheless, they occasionally occur. Those who get toothaches know how painful and impossible to tolerate they are. *Chamomilla* can help a person who is extremely sensitive to pain. For such people, one or two doses of three pellets of *Chamomilla* 30C can make a tremendous difference, both to help contain the pain and to help tolerate the drilling that is inevitably going to follow. Visits to a dentist would become so much easier if those who can't tolerate pain of any kind took it an hour before and immediately prior to visit.

When *Not* to Self-Medicate with *Chamomilla*

It is important to be mindful that angry children do not all require *Chamomilla*. If your child has significant behavioral problems, a visit to a homeopath is a good idea.

CHAPTER TWELVE

Gelsemium
Your Homeopathic Neurologist

"Some days it is a heroic act just to refuse the paralysis of fear and straighten up and step into another day."
—EDDIE ALBERT

Gelsemium sempervirens **(yellow jasmine, false jasmine, Carolina jessamine)** is one of the most useful homeopathic remedies we have for treating neurological disorders and acute anxiety. As you may recall from Chapter 8, it is also frequently used to treat the flu. All parts of the plant from which it is made are poisonous and cause gradual paralysis, which is the reason that it is required in cases where **symptoms develop gradually,** and why it is important in treating problems affecting the brain, spine, and nerves, including conditions such as motor paralysis of the eyes, throat, or limbs, multiple sclerosis, myasthenia gravis, and Parkinson's disease.

In cases that require Gelsemium, you will be able to see **significant weakness**, and neurological effects ranging from **tremors** to a **feeling of paralysis** (or even real paralysis).

The Origins of Gelsemium

Gelsemium sempervirens is one of the most beautiful native plants from the southern United States. According to Harvey Wickes Felter and John Uri Lloyd, authors of a nineteenth-century classic on medicinal herbs, *King's American Dispensatory*:

> *It is a twining vine, flourishing in great profusion from Virginia to Florida, hanging in festoons from the neighboring trees and shrubs, sometimes growing to the height of fifty feet. The average height, however, is from twenty to thirty feet. The plant blooms in early spring—in Florida during March, and in Mississippi and Tennessee in May and June. During the flowering period it perfumes the air with a delightful fragrance similar to that of the true jasmine. When the vine is abundant, the odor of the flowers is said to be almost overpowering.*[1]

Nicknamed false jasmine to distinguish it from true jasmine, which belongs to the family *Oleacea,* Gelsemium is classified as a member of the *Loganacea* family. Leafy and flowering parts of the plant are frequently used to decorate homes and gardens. However all parts of *Gelsemium sempervirens* are toxic, including the flower and the nectar. Highly poisonous, only its root is used in the preparation of the homeopathic remedy. True jasmine is native to Asia, not poisonous at all, and its flowers are used in jasmine tea and other herbal teas, and in blended black teas.

In 1753, the Carolina jessamine plant was originally identified and named *Bignonia sempervirens* by Swedish naturalist Carl Linnaeus. French botanist Antoine Laurent de Jussieu, whose subsequent work a few decades later piloted modern plant classification, renamed the genus in 1789. For this purpose, he changed the Italian word *gelsemino*, meaning "jasmine," into its Latin form. *Sempervirens* means "evergreen."

King's American Dispensatory offers the following description of the discovery of the medicinal qualities of Gelsemium:

> *This plant was brought into notice, as far as we can learn, in the following manner: A planter of Mississippi, whose name we have forgotten, while laboring under a severe attack of bilious fever, which resisted all the usual remedies, sent a servant into his garden to procure a certain medicinal root, and prepare an infusion of it for him to drink. The servant, by mistake, collected another root, and gave an infusion of it to his master, who, shortly after swallowing some of it, was seized with a complete loss of muscular power, unable to move a limb, or even raise his eyelids, although he could hear, and was cognizant of circumstances transpiring around him. His friends, greatly alarmed, collected around him, watching the result with much anxiety, and expecting every minute to see him breathe his last. After some hours, he gradually recovered himself, and was astonished to find that his fever had left him. Ascertaining from his servant what plant it was the root of which acted in this manner, he collected some of it, and employed it successfully on his own plantation, as well as among his neighbors. The success of this article finally reached the ear of some physician, who prepared from it a nostrum called the "Electrical Febrifuge," which was disguised with the essence of wintergreen. This plant was the yellow jessamine,*

and a knowledge of its remarkable effects was not communicated to the profession until a later period.[2]

If you read *National Geographic* or watch movies about Africa, you are probably noticing that the symptoms of yellow jasmine poisoning remind you of the effects of curare. You are correct. Curare and gelsemium belong to the same family of plants. So do St. Ignatius' bean and Quaker's buttons, the principle ingredients in the homeopathic remedies (*Ignatia amara* and *Nux vomica*) covered in the next two chapters. Another important member of the same family, *Spigelia*, will make an appearance in this chapter when we talk about the treatment of headaches.

Believing this family of plants is special because it has so many representatives amongst homeopathic remedies would be wrong. Numerous plant families provide important homeopathic remedies. This book would have to be a few thousand pages long to tell you about each and every one of them. Here we are presenting you with a few that can become your family's biggest allies in the course of everyday life.

The earliest descriptions of the homeopathic remedy prepared from *Gelsemium sempervirens* were published by American homeopaths in the 1850s and 1860s.

Symptoms Characteristic of the Gelsemium State

The key to understanding *Gelsemium* is that, when taken in its raw form, it affects the nervous system and, as a result, the person feels intoxicated, weak, and paralyzed. Therefore, any condition that begins with the following unique set of symptoms can be helped with homeopathically prepared *Gelsemium*.

- **Gradual onset.** Symptoms "creep up" on a person, like they do in cases of gradual paralysis
- Intoxicated feeling. Chills going up and down the spine. Weak and weary, cannot think
- Apathetic. Wants to be alone
- **Stage fright** (anticipation anxiety)
- The person is weak and lethargic. May even tremble from weakness
- Numbness
- **Eyelids feel heavy,** difficult to open
- Blurred vision
- Headache and **heaviness, mostly in the back of the head**

Conditions that trigger this combination of symptoms may include:
- Exposure to viruses.
- Performance.
- Neurological disorders (you need to see a neurologist as well as a homeopath to help these in the long run).

Things that make it feel worse include:
- Heat.
- **Warm and wet weather.**
- Cold and damp weather.
- Anticipation.
- Lying with head low.

Things that make it feel better are:
- **Profuse perspiration or urination.**
- Vomiting.
- Lying with head high.
- Alcohol (in cases of anxiety).
- Closing eyes.

Acute Anxiety

Gelsemium is an excellent remedy for stage fright and test anxiety. People who need this remedy to perform better under various circumstances literally feel paralyzed, weak, and dizzy. They tremble and fear losing control. Their limbs become heavy. This is not a good bouquet of symptoms to have during performances or exams.

For students coping with test anxiety, I recommend first trying out *Gelsemium* on an occasion when the stakes are lower and consequences seem less important, such as before a weekly quiz, rather than a midterm exam or a final. Imagine you were relying on a remedy to relieve your severe anxiety during an important test or a job interview and it didn't work. That could trigger more anxiety.

If *Gelsemium* does not bring relief, the next important remedy to consider is *Argentum nitricum* (see a description below).

Table 12.1 Acute Anxiety Remedy Comparison Chart

Remedy	Main Issues	Better from
Aconitum	Panic with no reason or after witnessing a horrific event; fear of doctors, dentists, surgery	Getting out of narrow place (bus, car, elevator)
Argentum nitricum	Anticipation anxiety (stage fright)	Motion; open air; company; talking
Gelsemium	Anticipation anxiety; terror before performance	Being alone

The protocol that I use is to take three pellets of *Gelsemium* 30C on the morning of the exam. I also prepare *Gelsemium* using the plussing method (see Chapter 3). The examinee takes a water bottle full of the diluted remedy to the test and sips from it as needed. You should not repeat the dose unless the anxiety begins to creep back on you. Each time you need to administer another dose, just shake the bottle again and drink about a teaspoon of the water. There's no need to add more pellets.

Exams are not the only anxiety-producing situation. Going on a date, especially for a shy person, can be an extreme emotional challenge. Another common cause of anxiety is public speaking. A few years ago, a family practice resident I was supervising told me that she felt so anxious speaking in public that she got weak and even trembled when she did. She asked for advice on what to do to prepare herself to give a wedding toast the next weekend. The miracle of *Gelsemium* turned her on to homeopathy.

Worse from	Guiding Signs	Remedy to Compare with
Narrow places; big crowds	Severe panic with fear of imminent death; loss of control; restlessness; feeling of being hot	*Argentum*
Warmth; being indoors	Hurried, nervous, always hot; desire for company and talking; afraid to be late; impulsive; has a sweet tooth	*Aconitum; Gelsemium*
Bad news; company	Timid; reserved; wants to be quiet	*Argentum*

If you have a tendency to become anxious, or suffer from anxiety disorder, a visit to a homeopath is a very good idea. On the other hand, I have seen cases when one time use of *Gelsemium*, or other remedy listed below, solved the issue of anxiety. Just be honest with yourself. If your problem continues, seek professional help.

Here are two other frequently indicated alternatives for cases of acute anxiety.

Aconitum napellus **(monkshood):** Indications of this state include:
- **Panic with fear of death.**
- Sudden panic attacks.
- **Loses control, becomes extremely restless.**
- **Needs to get out now** (for example, from an elevator or a subway car).
- Hyperventilation with tingling and numbness in the body.
- **Feels hot.**

Argentum nitricum **(silver nitrate):** Easily confused with *Gelsemium,* some experts suggest distinguishing the need for this remedy on the basis of diarrhea or other physical symptoms. Unfortunately, it is not always easy. However, there are certain features that make making the correct choice possible. Whereas someone in a *Gelsemium* state feels paralyzed from anxiety, an *Argentum nitricum* state is driven by anxiety on every level, including anxious diarrhea. People in a *Gelsemium* state want to be left alone. Those who need *Argentum nitricum* seek company and like to talk.

My advice to you in case of stage fright: when in doubt, start with *Gelsemium.*

Characteristic symptoms of *Argentum nitricum* are:
- Hurried, nervous.

- Fears: **being late,** closed spaces, heights (sometimes with impulse to jump).
- Wants company, talking.
- Has a sweet tooth.
- Worse from warmth, being indoors.
- Better from motion, open air.

Fatigue and Weakness

Most of us have been tired at some point of our life. If the feeling of exhaustion is a result of not having enough sleep, working too hard, not eating well these issues must be addressed. Homeopathy won't help. Stimulants might keep you up a bit longer, but ultimately you'll have to get enough sleep, food, and rest if you want to feel better.

Another side of exhaustion and fatigue is a possible underlying illness such as COVID-19, common colds and flu, mononucleosis, Lyme disease, diabetes, liver disorders, and thyroid conditions. The list may go on and on. The bottom line is to seek rest, sleep, and food if there was a lack of them. If there wasn't such a deficit, or you don't feel restored soon after taking self-care measures, go see a physician. In cases when the reason for exhaustion is identified and it isn't due to a significant illness, *Gelsemium* may be of great assistance.

Gelsemium should be considered if fatigue sets in after a viral infection and also in cases of feeling weak from fear, anticipation, or prolonged mental effort. (Compare this to *Picricum acidum.*) A person who needs *Gelsemium* feels drowsy and dull, and has muscular weakness and trembling. The back of the head and limbs feel heavy. This individual wants to be left alone—completely alone, even a quiet person is unwelcome in the same room. The condition is made worse by heat.

Below are six other frequently helpful remedies for fatigue. You'll notice that the last three are acids. Homeopathic remedies made from acids share one pronounced characteristic: They help reduce weakness from different types of causes. Every time a practitioner sees someone whose main complaint is weakness, then the first possible remedy matches that come to mind are *Gelsemium* and the acids.

Of the most frequently indicated homeopathic acids *Muriaticum acidum* is indicated mostly for people who experience physical weakness, *Picricum acidum* for people who feel weak after prolonged intellectual strain, such as cramming for exams or finishing a book, and *Phosphoricum acidum* for those who become weak and feel indifferent after enduring a severe emotional strain, such as grief.

Please remember that a person who becomes extremely weak after hearing bad news most probably needs *Gelsemium*. In cases such as these, you'll also see all the other typical identifying characteristics of the state, including a headache.

Let's look at the six common alternatives to *Gelsemium* now.

***Arsenicum album* (oxide of arsenic):** Indications of this state are:
- Weakness with anxiety and restlessness.
- Feeling chilled.
- **Having burning pains that are better from heat.**
- Very fastidious, becomes very organized in a kind of neurotic, anxious way.
- Insecure, fear of death.
- Thirsty for small sips of cold water.
- Worse from cold and drinking alcoholic beverages. (Compare to *Gelsemium*, which is better from alcohol.)
- Better from heat and company. (Gelsemium wants to be left alone.)

Carbo vegetabilis **(vegetable charcoal):** Indications of this state are:
- Fainting in public places due to being exhausted.
- Must have fresh air.
- **Better from fanning** or direct flow from air conditioning.

China (Cinchona officinalis): Indications of this state are:
- **Extreme exhaustions after blood loss, anemia or prolonged illness.**
- Periodic symptoms (every hour, every day, every other day, and so on).
- Acute senses, hypersensitive to touch, or even a current of air, but tolerates continuous pressure well.
- Vertigo.
- Tinnitus (various sounds in the ear).
- Bitter taste in the mouth, and even food that is desired tastes bitter.
- Worse from motion.

Muriaticum acidum **(hydrochloric acid):** Considered one of the best remedies for typhoid fever, which is characterized by severe weakness. Other indications are:
- **Weakness on the physical rather than the emotional level**, exhaustion from clear physical reasons.
- Severe weakness after, or even during a long illness with high temperature.
- Extremely crabby and weak.
- Involuntary stool when passing urine.
- Protruding hemorrhoids.
- Worse: lying on the right side, sea bathing.

Table 12.2 Fatigue and Weakness Remedy Comparison Chart

Remedy	Better	Worse
Arsenicum	Heat; company	Cold; alcohol
Carbo vegetabilis	Fanning	Stuffy room
China	Open air; warmth	Slightest touch; air; night
Gelsemium	Profuse urination; open air; continued motion	Time preceding a thunderstorm; damp weather; excitement; 10 AM
Muriaticum acidum	Lying on the left side	Lying on the right side; sea bathing
Phosphoricum acidum	Keeping warm; juicy fruit	Being talked to; sex; loss of vital fluids
Picricum acidum	Cold air; cold water	Even the slightest mental exertion

Emotional State	Signs Guiding Your Selection	Remedy to Compare with
Anxious; restless; afraid of illnesses and death	Insecurity combined with fastidiousness; neurotic behavior; thirst for small sips of cold water	*China; Gelsemium*
Disoriented	Fainting in public places from exhaustion	*China; Gelsemium*
Sensitive to noise; touchy; afraid of animals (even pets); has many thoughts at night before going to sleep	Exhaustion after massive blood loss or any other fluid loss e.g., prolonged diarrhea)	*Gelsemium*
Timid; reserved; want to be alone	Weakness that increases gradually; difficulties opening the eyes	*China; Phosphoricum; Muriaticum*
Simply exhausted; no specific emotional features	Weakness that is purely physical; extreme crabbiness and weakness; involuntary stool while urinating	*Gelsemium; Phosphoricum*
Grieving; forgetful after grief; indifferent; lifeless; apathetic; feels dead inside	Weakness from grief or after a prolonged illness (e.g., mononucleosis)	*China; Gelsemium; Muriaticum*
Aversion to thinking, talking, or doing anything at all; Often says, "I can't think."	Exhaustion after intense mental work (e.g., cramming for exams or finishing a project or a book)	*Phosphoricum*

***Phosphoricum acidum* (phosphoric acid):** Indications of this state are:
- **Weakness from grief.**
- **Forgetful, mental weakness after grief.**
- Also weakness after prolonged illness (for example, mononucleosis or prolonged diarrhea) or after drug and alcohol abuse.
- Lifeless, apathetic, as if dead inside.
- Hair become gray, or even fell off, while grieving.
- Craves fruit, juices, refreshing foods.
- **Paradoxically may have profuse diarrhea without expected weakness.**

***Picricum acidum* (picric acid):** Indications of this state are:
- **Exhaustion after long studies (such as cramming for exams) or prolonged intellectual strain.**
- Indifference.
- Aversion to doing anything, even thinking or talking. Frequently people in this state say: "I cannot think."

Headaches and Migraines

Treatment of chronic cluster and migraine headaches is a definite forte of homeopathy. The remedies in this section will help to eliminate your pain during an acute headache or the worsening of a chronic condition. But if your goal is to cure your headaches, rather than manage or ease them, it will be best to consult a homeopath. Prior to going to a homeopath you should most definitely address the issue of having a chronic headache with a neurologist and, if necessary with a doctor who specializes in the treatment of chronic headaches. Safety first.

See a homeopath only after you learned that there are no diagnosable reasons for your headaches that can be easily addressed by conventional medicine. The reason some remedies are listed here is that these have clear and unique characteristics. If you happen to know someone whose headaches include these symptoms, or if they are characteristic of your own headaches, you are fortunate indeed. A remedy taken for acute pain may wind up curing the entire problem.

There are a few things that a migraine or headache sufferer could do in addition to taking homeopathy. For example:

1. **An elimination diet.** Food allergies have been shown to be one of the major triggers of migraine headaches.[3] Undergoing the process of an elimination diet for a few weeks can help you to understand whether or not you are suffering from food allergies. To do an elimination diet, you remove individual foods from your diet for a period of time, such as a week, and then return to eating them in a large quantity for one day. If you are sensitive to a particular food, you will experience noticeable symptoms then.

2. **Abstaining from coffee.** Some people benefit from eating regular meals and abstaining from coffee and other foods and beverages containing caffeine.

3. **Taking the herb feverfew.** Feverfew is a popular herbal treatment for headaches. Some people swear by it, and research has shown it to be effective.[4] Feverfew does not interfere with homeopathic treatment.

4. **Bodywork.** Other effective nonhomeopathic measures for treating headaches include craniosacral therapy and acupuncture. But you should know that some homeopaths (yours truly included) feel that acupuncture interferes with homeopathic treatment.

5. **Over-the-counter nonsteroidal anti-inflammatory (NSAID) medication.** Many headache sufferers routinely take three to four tablets of aspirin, acetaminophen (for example, Tylenol), or ibuprofen (for example, Motrin or Advil) for each episode of headache. Be forewarned that there is a phenomenon known as a rebound headache in which a vicious cycle is created of headache-medication-rebound headache-more medication, and so on.

Warning: See a physician if a headache is unusual or extreme. Let me warn you again, more explicitly. If somebody who has never or rarely had a headache suddenly develops a severe headache, getting a full medical workup ASAP is indicated. The same is true for someone who develops repeated headaches. Go see the doctor. Better safe than sorry.

Gelsemium helps severe, exhausting headaches that show these signs.

- Heaviness in the head (**especially if it begins in the back and extends to the forehead**) or a sensation of having a tight band around the head
- Difficult to hold head straight
- Difficult to open the eyes
- **Blurred vision or double vision during the headache**
- **Severe weakness with trembling during the headache**
- Worse: 10 AM, lying flat
- Better: **urination** (especially profuse urination), lying with elevated head

Additional remedies for acute headaches include:

Arnica montana **(leopard's bane):** Should always be considered first for headaches after a head trauma. Indications of this state include:
- Wanting to be left alone.
- Better from lying down flat with head low.
- Worse from waking up before 10 AM.

Calcarea phosphorica **(calcium phosphate):** If this is the right remedy, I recommend using a cell salt in 6X potency. *Instructions*: Take three to five tablets, two to three times a day for a month. Important characteristics are:

- **Headaches in schoolchildren that come after lunch or the end of the school day.**
- Usually the headache is combined with a stomachache.

China (Chinchona officinalis): Indications of this state include:

- **Headaches after a serious loss of fluids, as for example happens during prolonged menopausal bleeding, breastfeeding, diarrhea, or such as are associated with anemia.**
- Weakness.
- Pain is the whole head and goes into teeth.
- Pale during the headache.
- Feeling that the brain hits the walls of the inside of the skull.
- Worse: from open air, drafts, noise, motion, and even touch.
- Better: from **hard pressure** with hand, warm room, moving head up and down.

Cocculus indicus **(Indian cockle):** Indications of this state include:

- **Headache from many worries and loss of sleep,** as for example happens when taking care of a loved one who is very ill.
- Headache with dizziness, nausea and vomiting. Vomiting can be triggered by noise.
- Pain is frequently located in the back of the head (compare with *Gelsemium),* can also be in the whole head.
- Worse: from **riding in a car as a passenger, loss of sleep.**
- Better: from sleep, lying on a side.

Table 12.3 General Headaches and Migraines Remedy Comparison Chart

Remedy	Better	Worse
Arnica	Lying down with head low	Waking up until 10 AM
Calcarea phosphorica	Warm, dry weather	Change of weather; after lunch or at the end of the day
China	Hard pressure with hand; moving head up and down; warm room; hot weather	Lying flat; 10 AM
Cocculus	Sleep; lying on the side (takes pressure off the back of the head)	Loss of sleep; riding in a car; lying on the back; pressure on the back of the head
Gelsemium	Urination; lying down with head elevated	Time preceding a thunderstorm; damp weather; excitement; 10 AM
Ignatia	Lying on painful side; alcohol; motion; warm applications	Emotions; being in a room where other people smoke
Nux vomica	Warm applications; lying on the painless side; morning (rising from bed)	Cold; alcohol; noise; light; morning in bed

Emotional State	Signs Guiding Your Selection	Remedy to Compare with
Wants to be left alone	Headaches after head trauma	
Peevish; always wants change, to go somewhere	Headaches in schoolchildren	
Sensitive to noise; touchy	Headaches after significant fluid loss (prolonged bleeding, prolonged diarrhea, etc.) or anemia	*Gelsemium*
Sensitive and sympathetic; anxious about loved ones	Headaches from worries (e.g., as a result of taking care of a sick relative or friend)	*Gelsemium*
Timid; reserved; wants to be alone	Heaviness that begins in the back of the head and travels to the forehead; difficulties opening the eyes	*China; Cocculus*
Easily hurt; easily offended; may be hysterical	Headaches after grief, divorce, or breakup; pain that feels like a nail was stuck in the side of the4 head	*Cocculus*
Irritable and very easily offended (characteristics are magnified during the headache)	Headaches from hangover, drug abuse, and tension; migraine headaches	*Ignatia*

Ignatia amara **(St. Ignatius' bean):** Indications of this state include:
- **Headaches caused by bad news** (e.g., a breakup) and grief.
- Headache with back or neck spasms.
- Pain feels **like a nail** was stuck in the side of head.

Nux vomica **(poison nut):** Indications of this state include:
- **Tension headaches as a result of a hangover, toxic headaches.**
- **Oversensitive to all stimuli.**
- **Irritable, angry.**
- Constipation during headache.
- Worse: from **cold**, stimuli (examples: noise, odor, light, wind), motion, eating, and lying on painful side (compare to *Bryonia*).
- Better: from **warm** applications, lying on painless side.

Right-Sided Headaches and Migraines

Our discussion would not be complete if we did not address remedies helpful for pain on a particular side of the head. Here are five remedies for right-sided pain.

Belladonna **(deadly nightshade):** Indications of this are:
- Headache starts or disappears suddenly (sometimes both).
- Extremely painful, **pulsating** headache. Sufferer may report that the pain is "exploding" or "maddening."
- Sensation that the brain is pressing **outward.** You may hear, "It feels like my eyes will pop out."
- Begins in the back of the head and either extends to the other side, or goes to the right forehead and/or the eye.
- Pupils are large.

- Head feels hot, face flushed; but hands and/or feet are cold.
- Worse from motion, light, noise, stooping, washing hair.
- Better from lying in a quiet, dark room.

Cedron (**cedron seed**): Indications of this state are:
- **Pain returns at exactly the same time**: same hour, every day, every three days, weekly, monthly, or so forth.
- Head feels swollen.
- Body feels numb during the headache.

Iris versicolor (**harlequin blueflag**):
- Frequently indicated for classical headaches that come on weekends, during rest.
- **Headache begins with visual aura and ends with vomiting.**
- **Blurry vision, sometimes even blindness during headache** (compare with *Belladonna*).
- Headache may go from side to side.
- Worse from rest, sitting, cold air.
- Better from walking, standing, constant relaxed motion.

Ranunculus bulbosus (**St. Anthony's turnip**): Indications of this state are:
- Headache before a storm.
- Alcohol makes it much worse.

Sanguinaria canadensis (**bloodroot**): Indications of this state are:
- **Headache begins in the back of the head, or even neck and shoulder, and goes into the right eye.**
- Face is flushed with pulsating carotids (compare carefully to *Belladonna*).

Table 12.4 Right-Sided Headaches Remedy Comparison Chart

Remedy	Better	Worse
Belladonna	Lying in a quiet, dark room	Light; sound
Cedron	No modalities	Rising; open air; 9 AM or 11 AM
Iris	Constant slow, relaxed motion; standing	Rest; sitting; cold air
Ranunculus	Standing or walking	Time preceding a storm; change of weather; alcohol
Sanguinaria	Vomiting; sleep or rest; pressing head against hard surfaces	Fasting; daytime (comes and goes with the sun)

Emotional State	Signs Guiding Your Selection	Remedy to Compare with
Acute sense; sensitive to light and sound	Extreme painfulness; maddening, pulsating headache (as if brain is pressing outward and as if the eyes will pop out)	*Iris*
No specific data	Pain that comes back at exactly the same hour (daily, every two days, ort any periodicity); possible numbness of the whole body along with the headache	*Sanguinaria*
No specific data	Classic migraine that begins with aura and ends with vomiting; blindness during the headache	*belladonna*
Irritable	Headache that starts before a storm; headache that is much worse from alcohol; (can be triggered by alcohol)	*Sanguinaria*
No specific data	Pain that begins in the back of the head, frequently in the neck and shoulder, and then goes into the eye; menopausal headaches; flushed face with pulsating carotids	*Belladonna*

Table 12.5 Left-Sided Headaches Remedy Comparison Chart

Remedy	Better	Worse
Bryonia	Immobilization; pressure; lying on the painful side	The slightest motion (even of the eyes or of the eyelids closing and opening)
Sepia	Vigorous exercise; eating	Time before and/or during menses; sex (in contrast to most people who report improvement of headaches during sex)
Spigelia	Heat (e.g., a hot bath); lying down with head elevated and eyes closed	Any exertion, even straining to pass a stool; jarring; cold; open air

- Headaches appears with the sunrise and goes away with the sunset.
- Vomiting during headaches.
- Periodic headaches.
- Worse during the daytime and from light, noise, odors, fasting, jarring, and menses.
- Better from sleep, rest, after vomiting, and pressing head against hard surfaces.

Left-Sided Headaches

To balance out the last section, here are remedies specifically for left-sided pain.

Emotional State	Signs Guiding Your Selection	Remedy to Compare with
Irritable; wants to be alone	Pain that is much worse from motion; pain that begins over the left eye and goes into the back and spreads over the entire head	*Spigelia*
Wants to be alone	Better from exercise and eating; clearly worse around menses	*Spigelia*
Possibly afraid of sharp objects	Pain that is exactly above the left eye	*Bryonia; Sepia*

Bryonia alba **(white bryony):** Indications of this state are:
- Bursting headache that begins over the left eye and goes into the back of the head. May spread to the entire head.
- Headache starts in the morning, or at 9 PM.
- Worse from **even a slight motion** (like moving eyes, or closing and opening eyelids).
- Better from pressure (because nothing can be moved), lying on a painful side (same idea of not moving).

Sepia **(cuttle fish ink):** Indications of this state are:
- Headache is in the left forehead or above the left eye (compare with *Spigelia*).
- "Sick headache" (with nausea).

- Worse **before and/or during the period**, from sex (most migraine sufferers report improvement during sex or masturbation), and artificial lighting.
- Better from **vigorous exercise** (compare with many other remedies; most are worse from motion), and **eating.**

Spigelia **(pinkroot):** Indications of this state are:
- **Above the left eye.**
- Violent pain in one spot that the person can clearly point with one finger.
- The pain is like a **stitch in the side.**
- Headache may be associated with heart palpitations beat or any other heart problems.
- Worse from jarring, any type of exertion, including straining to pass a stool, cold, open air, wind, and smoke.
- Better from heat, taking a hot bath, and lying with elevated head and closed eyes.

A Few Other Conditions That May Require *Gelsemium*

Some people develop significant signs of anxiety when they have diarrhea, and show all the typical modalities of *Gelsemium* on those occasions. *Gelsemium* is also helpful in many cases of fever and flu. As a matter of fact, as you already learned in Chapter 8, *Gelsemium* is one of the main remedies used for the treatment of flu.

When *Not* to Self-Medicate with *Gelsemium*

You may be asking: But what about all the neurological conditions such as tremors, multiple sclerosis, myasthenia gravis, and paralysis? *Gelsemium* is one of many remedies that may relieve the suffering of the victims of all these diseases, but the patient needs to follow up with a neurologist and a homeopath to address treatment of this chronic conditions.

My mother had a pretty dramatic experience with *Gelsemium.* One beautiful winter morning she woke up with a significant fever and weakness. She also had a headache that featured tremendous heaviness in the back of her head. I was at work all day and by the time I got home my independent-minded mother had taken some aspirin. Her fever was down a bit, but the weakness continued to worsen.

By the end of the evening, my mother was having difficulties opening her eyes. Actually, one eye was completely closed. Knowing that she had been suffering from hypertension and that both of her parents died from strokes, my father suggested that perhaps we should take her to the hospital. There we ascertained that her fever was not an issue anymore. The doctor in the ER decided to rule out two of the most serious possibilities—a ministroke and myasthenia gravis, an illness that might present itself through drooping of the eye—so my mother was hospitalized.

The moment my mother was settled in her room, I gave her a few pellets of *Gelsemium* 30C. After all, you and I understand that the big picture of the combination of all her symptoms was pointing to this remedy. The next morning, her headache was gone, she felt stronger, and her eyes could open. Of course, she was in a hospital setting. All the tests were done and we played it very safe. But the fact remains that *Gelsemium* saved the day.

Why didn't I give it to her right away? Try taking care of a stubborn older mother yourself and then get back to me on this one.

CHAPTER THIRTEEN

Ignatia
Your Homeopathic
Therapist

"Where Joy most Revels, Grief doth most lament;
Grief joys, Joy grieves on slender accident."
—WILLIAM SHAKESPEARE, *HAMLET*

*I*gnatia amara **(St. Ignatius' bean, *Strychnos ignatii*)** is one of the most commonly needed remedies for coping with grief and loss. It provides relief by healing emotional pain and physical complaints that result from bereavement. You'll know that *Ignatia* is the right remedy if the person who takes it feels that the situation they are mourning remains real, as if it happened yesterday, and continues constantly to focus on it.

The value of this remedy in modern society cannot be overestimated. It is used to treat both the initial stages and the long-term consequences of emotional crises, such as a divorce, a miscarriage, a sudden job loss, and the death of a close friend, witnessing the devastation of war, or moving away from home. Today we are becoming ever more aware of the effects of various psychological issues like these, as going to a therapist is now as routine as visiting a local pastry shop was one hundred years ago. Therefore, we have more experience in overcoming such losses. *Ignatia* comes in handy in all these types of situations, and can improve your resilience so you and your family members don't get stuck in the past.

How can you recognize the *Ignatia amara* state? *Ignatia* is a medication for grief and anguish. Among other traits, the person who needs this remedy has hysterical reactions, like prolonged crying jags and numbness. Another important feature of the state it cures is that it includes paradoxical behavior, such as an upset person refusing to be consoled and comforted; and counterintuitive symptoms, such as throat pain that's improved, rather than worsened, by the act of swallowing.

The Origins of Ignatia

Strychnos ignatii, the botanical name for the plant from which this remedy is derived, is a large, woody, climbing shrub that produces large, extremely bitter fruit. Resembling a medium-sized pear, the fruit has seeds that are about an inch long. As you may have guessed, the fruit's bitterness is due to strychnine contained in the seeds, which makes them poisonous on one hand and of high medicinal value on the other. Homeopathic preparations are made from the seeds.

The plant is indigenous to the Philippine Islands, where the natives have long recognized its therapeutic properties. But instead of preparing potions from it, they wore the seeds as amulets for the prevention and cure of various diseases. Malaysians call ignatia *upas paja,* meaning "royal poison," and historically used the juice of the fruit to poison their arrows for hunting, and occasionally to murder their human enemies.

The Europeans learned about ignatia from Spanish priests who named the shrub after the founder of the Jesuit Order, Ignatius Loyola.

Jesuit priest George Kamel, a man who dedicated his life to natural science, collected the plant and introduced the seed known as St. Ignatius' bean to Europe in the latter half of the seventeenth century.

In 1818, French chemists Joseph Caventou and Pierre-Joseph Pelletier discovered strychnine while studying the contents of St. Ignatius' bean. Interestingly, both *Ignatia amara* and *Nux vomica,* a plant scientifically known as *Strychnos nux-vomica* and colloquially called either Quaker buttons or poison fruit (see Chapter 12), contain strychnine and another alkaloid, brucine, however in different proportions. Ignatia contains one third more strychnine and a lesser percentage of brucine than nux vomica does.

Samuel Hahnemann conducted the first proving of the remedy Ignatia amara and described it in great detail. As in the many other cases we've discussed, his discovery of the innovative homeopathic method for the preparation of remedies allowed him to extract the medicinal qualities of this amazing plant and neutralize its poisonous qualities.

Symptoms Characteristic of the *Ignatia* State

Many homeopathic authorities have written that *Ignatia* is the "female counterpart" of *Nux vomica,* which is considered by some a remedy "for males." This comparison is tempting, because both remedies are derived from plants that belong to the same genus, *Strychnos*. The idea of male and female attributes complementing each other in nature has always been enticing to humankind. Although it may be true, the reality of the modern lifestyle is that in their routine daily existence people of both genders who benefit from taking *Ignatia* are sensitive, easily excitable, and "quick in perceiving, prompt in appreciation and rapid in execution."¹ These people are also **highly idealistic** and **really** don't appreciate contradiction.

As we all know, our era is characterized by globalization and integration. This trend certainly affects the way men and women think, feel, and behave. Contrary to the historical record, in my practice I have seen many men who benefited from *Ignatia* and many women who were cured by *Nux vomica*.

An even more important concept to appreciate is that at certain ages and under the influence of certain situations people have a tendency to move into particular mental, emotional, and physical states. After reading this chapter, you'll be able to see that going through adolescence and being romantically involved and then losing a close person both may move a person into the condition that can be remedied by *Ignatia*.

An essential detail to recognize is that **people who need *Ignatia* feel as if they lost someone just a few hours earlier.** The wound is still fresh. The emotional pain is acute—even if the loss happened a long time ago. It's as if whomever they are missing was just here, and is only now gone. And the loss feels terribly unfair. The pain is practically unbearable!

Later in the chapter, when you read about the picture of *Natrum muriaticum,* the "twin" of *Ignatia* from the mineral kingdom, keep in mind that this sense of experiencing a fresh and painful loss is the main feature distinguishing it from *Ignatia*.

The state that requires *Ignatia* can best be described in one word: *hysteria*. According to one medical dictionary, "Hysteria [is] excessive or uncontrollable emotion."² When people are hysterical, it doesn't mean they are exceedingly amused, as in the phrase *laughing hysterically,* it means people are feeling and acting out of control.

A lot of symptoms in the *Ignatia* state seem to be exactly the opposite of what you'd expect. For example, there may be a fever but no thirst, a sore throat that is improved by swallowing, sensitivity that is relieved by pressure, a chill offset by removing covers, a headache relieved by the act of bending forward, and so on. This tendency for reversal is so pronounced that Andrew L. Monroe, M.D., a prominent American homeopath of the nineteenth century, once said: "One must look for the body of a drowned Ignatia patient 'up stream.'"[3]

People who need *Ignatia* don't necessarily act crazy; rather, these individuals usually feel like things are going out of control and they must do everything they can to control themselves. Not always successful in this regard, sometimes they do achieve it.

Let's look at prominent examples of symptoms caused by the effort to control yourself despite the feeling that things are literally falling apart, as you might feel in the case of being abandoned by a loved one either due to death or a relationship breakup. Those who need *Ignatia* might:

- Have a *globus* hystericus—a medical term for feeling a "lump" in the throat.
- Attempt to suppress crying and wind up sobbing.
- Dislike sympathy and consolation because someone might see how devastated they really are. Teenagers, for instance, frequently run into their bedrooms, lock the door behind them, and then start crying uncontrollably.
- Sigh, because the chest tightens up from their effort to keep the emotions inside.
- Experience numbness, or even temporary paralysis, without a physical cause. This is also caused by trying to hold everything inside.
- Have back spasms from stress-related tension after grief. (Do you get it now?)
- Be very defensive, touchy, and easily offended.

- Want to travel and feel much better when traveling. They have a desire to escape and hide their real emotions.

Circumstances that trigger this combination of symptoms may include:
- The death of a loved one or a companion animal.
- A breakup or divorce.
- A miscarriage.
- Being the victim of a violent act, such as an assault, rape, or robbery.
- Being the victim of an accident or another scary event.
- For children, watching their parents fighting or getting a divorce.
- Homesickness.
- Unfair treatment.
- Being fired from a job.

Let's talk about specific situations in which *Ignatia* and a few other remedies can be of great help. You may notice that there are only a few additional remedies described here; less than in the other chapters. The reason is simple: The emotional core is the most complicated and sophisticated part of a human being. Only a few remedies with the most obvious symptoms are appropriate for self-care. Fortunately, these are the remedies people often tend to need.

More complicated grieving situations should be treated by an experienced homeopath, and it is highly desirable to involve a mental health professional in the treatment plan. I am qualified as both a psychiatrist and a homeopath.

Emotional Crisis and Grief

As you can probably imagine, in my medical practice I've had to prescribe *Ignatia* on numerous occasions. The following two case studies will serve to illustrate the key symptoms and remarkable curative power of this great remedy.

Once I treated a young woman suffering from bipolar disorder. In the initial interview to evaluate her, she told me she wasn't doing well on her conventional medications and therefore was looking to improve the quality of her life using complementary methods of treatment. After an hour together, it was clear that my patient needed *Ignatia* for constitutional treatment of her condition. Before she left, I gave her a dose of three pellets of *Ignatia amara* 200C and we decided to meet again a month later.

Our follow-up appointment started with the woman describing how amazingly easy it was for her to tolerate her latest breakup. Her boyfriend of more than a year had ended their relationship three days after our first meeting. Prior to taking *Ignatia,* breakups like this one—even those that she herself initiated—were always devastating to my patient, and would send her into a deep depression. This time, she reported, "I was hurt, but it was more on the intellectual, rather than emotional level. I was absolutely fine!"

I have had to prescribe *Ignatia* for broken hearts on many occasions. It does miracles both prophylactically and after the event, but only under one condition: that the person who takes it is demonstrating typical symptoms of this remedy. Taking *Ignatia* before a traumatic event works only for people—usually girls and women—who have a tendency to suffer at the end of relationships. Still, it is worth keeping *Ignatia amara* 200C on hand just in case it is ever needed.

Another situation where *Ignatia* is frequently of great help is grief following a death. I have lost a few people with whom I was close in my life. So far, the most painful experience was at the death of my eighty-seven-year-old father. But I didn't need the remedy, my mother did. Taking *Ignatia* literally changed her entire attitude, not only immediately after the fact but also when we went to visit the grave for the first time after the burial. A few other elderly women who came along on this occasion also benefited greatly.

Instructions: Please take all remedies for emotional crisis and grief in concentration 200C, three pellets at a time. *Ignatia amara* 200C can be taken as needed for the duration of an emotional crisis, provided that it produces the effect of lessening the severity of your emotional strain. *Ignatia* is the most useful homeopathic remedy for coping with acute grief and it is indicated in a large proportion of cases.

Of course, *Ignatia* is far from a one-size-fits-all proposition. Below you will find descriptions of two other remedies that are frequently required for emotional crises and grief. Always compare *Ignatia* with *Natrum muriaticum* and *Phosphoricum acidum*, and especially the latter. If you are having the correct symptoms, I recommend taking either *Natrum muriaticum* or *Phosphoricum acidum* only once. *Dose*: Three 200C pellets. These remedies are long acting and will work just fine after a single dose.

If you happen to take a dose or two of the wrong remedy when you're in an emotional crisis, no harm will be done, however it is a good idea to proceed with seeing a professional homeopath in order to gain some relief. There is no need to suffer.

Natrum muriaticum (sodium chloride): The picture of this remedy can be difficult to distinguish from the picture of *Ignatia*. But there is one major distinction: People who need *Ignatia* are usually idealistic, trusting, and high energy. If something bad happens, they are disillusioned and totally unprepared for the loss, and therefore go into the *Ignatia* state. As I mentioned before, *Ignatia* is indicated when the loss feels as if it happened a few hours ago, or like it was "just yesterday." People needing *Natrum muriaticum* are different. They are born to be sensitive to any loss. It is their nature to look back in the past. For this reason, homeopaths frequently use the biblical story of Lot's wife from Genesis as a metaphor for people who need *Natrum muriaticum*.

As the story goes, God gave Lot and his immediate family an opportunity to escape the destruction of Sodom and Gomorrah. The only stipulation of their salvation was that they weren't allowed to watch—only to flee. Despite this warning, Lot's wife glanced backwards over her shoulder and was transformed into a pillar of salt. What is the raw material of *Natrum muriaticum?* Sodium chloride, or table salt!

Natrum muriaticum is usually beneficial to people who've been exposed to many losses and review them mentally. More importantly, those who need this remedy are extremely sensitive to loss, as someone might feel when relocating to a new town, or a teenager might feel whose friends were going to a different school. Another important tendency of people who need this remedy is trying to keep everything locked up inside. They do this more successfully than people who need *Ignatia*. Such a person is reserved, proper, and quiet even at an early age.

The chief characteristics of *Natrum muriaticum* are:
- **Too serious** (for example, children who are too serious for their age), proper, extremely responsible.
  - Likely to gain much relief—relaxation, laughter—from imbibing alcoholic drinks (this trait might lead to alcoholism and drug abuse).
  - Depressed, but cannot cry.
  - Easily offended, hurt.

Table 13.1 Emotional Crisis and Grief Remedy Comparison Chart

Remedy	Better	Worse
Ignatia	Traveling	Consolation
Natrum muriaticum	Alcohol; going without regular meals	Consolation; talking
Phosphoricum acidum	No data	Being talked to

- **Giggle while telling about sad stories** (for example, a girl who describes being abused by her mother and giggles as if it is funny).
- **Dwells on past losses and humiliations.**
- Perfectionism, dressing very neatly (even children).
- Being easily moved by music (to both tears and laughter). Loving music.
- **Unable to tolerate exposure to the sun.**
- **Migraine headaches.**
- Cold sores on the lips and, especially, inside of the mouth.

Emotional State	Signs Guiding Your Selection	Remedy to Compare with
Romantic disappointment; grief; defensive; touchy; easily offended	Grief that is very much on the surface (regardless of real time); tendency to be easily hurt and offended; possibly, rudeness and suspiciousness; sighing and sobbing	*Natrum muriaticum*
Reserved; very responsible; reliable	Sadness but with inability to cry; inclination to giggle while talking about very sad events; tendency to be easily moved by music; tendency for dwelling on past occurrences; craving for salt	*Ignatia*
Apathetic; feels frozen and dead inside	Depression; apathy; lifelessness; exhaustion due to grief	*Ignatia; Natrum muriaticum*

- **Back pain (frequently in the lower back) much improved from lying on a hard surface (for example a floor or a book).**
- **Craving salt.**

In an article in *Homeopathy Today,* the periodic journal of the National Center for Homeopathy, Todd A. Hoover, M.D., described the type of person needing *Natrum muriaticum* well: "These individuals are literally swollen with grief."[4] That sense of emotional "swelling" frequently translates into physical problems, which for instance might include severe migraine headaches. Natrum muriaticum relieves such ailments.

We shouldn't underestimate the power a single dose of the right remedy can have on us—or other living creatures. Homeopath Jack Lawyer told me the true story of Seri, a young elephant who at the time lived in the Rosemond Gifford Zoo in Syracuse, New York. She had a happy relationship with her keeper, Chuck, and frolicked happily in her enclosure, until he got promoted and couldn't have close contact with her anymore. This was a great shock to her. You could easily compare the impact on the elephant of this decision to the trauma people experience when they watch close relatives accidentally die. As a result, Seri experienced symptoms typical of post-traumatic stress disorder or depression: Seri lost interest in activities; she developed severe physical symptoms that included pain and swelling in her legs and ulcers on her ankles; and she became irritable and angry. She was so sad that she gradually withdrew and wouldn't interact with anyone. It enraged her if people tried to break into her solitude. Her appetite was also poor.

Zoo staff called veterinarians numerous times, but all their efforts to treat Seri using conventional veterinary medicine were in vain. The grief-stricken young elephant continued to suffer. In fact, she was literally dying. Finally, the staff saw only one way to relieve Seri of her misery: She had to be put down.

Although Anne Baker, the executive director of the zoo, didn't believe in homeopathy, she was a good friend of Jack, knew about his studies of homeopathy, and decided, as a last resort, to ask him what he thought they could do. Jack visited Seri. He noticed many important things about this elephant and gave her a dose of *Natrum muriaticum* 1M. This single dose of the remedy brought Seri back to life. After its administration she began gradually improving, and soon returned to being a happy elephant. Jack visited Seri many times, but he never saw the need to give her another dose of the remedy.[5]

Phosphoricum acidum **(phosphoric acid):** The best description I've ever heard of the emotional state that requires this remedy was one offered by eminent American homeopath Paul Herscu. Imagine a dog that lived with its owner for many years. One day the owner takes the dog to the airport, sits it in the corner, gets on a plane, and flies away forever. Meanwhile, the dog just sits there in total despair and waits. It doesn't move. It doesn't eat. It is so overwhelmed by the loss that it is simply unable to respond to anything else.

Like this sorrowful dog that has been so grievously abandoned, the person who needs *Phosphoricum acidum* feels completely drained of energy. The person is apathetic, enervated, and bone tired. In essence, the person feels dead. Someone can develop the state that requires this remedy as a result of loss or physical illnesses like mononucleosis or chronic diarrhea. In addition, alcohol and drug abuse frequently lead to a similar state.

Here are important characteristics of the remedy.

- Apathy
- **Forgetfulness.** Gets lost easily. Frequently reports developing problems with memory after grief.
- **Indifference.** Frequently just sits or lies around all day.
- **Craving juicy fruit, fruit juices, refreshing drinks**
- Better from sleep, even if it is a short nap.

Depression

On its own, any medication, even a powerful homeopathic remedy, cannot resolve the multiple issues a depressed person has. Combining homeopathy and psychotherapy is a significantly more beneficial approach. Of course, it is easier said than done if you decide to locate a psychiatrist who also knows homeopathy. My credentials, which unite these professions, are rare. However, if such a combination is not available near you, first connect with a good psychiatrist and then seek homeopathic help separately. Never attempt to treat depression yourself. Always seek help from a mental health professional.

Why would I recommend a homeopathic remedy if the person is going to the hospital? Because there is literally no conventional medication that treats suicidality. In fact, as you may be aware, the FDA issued recent warnings about the increase of suicidal behavior due to the use of conventional antidepressants. Although *Aurum metallicum* isn't the only possible remedy for suicidal people, it is the most frequently indicated one. It will do its job in the long run. I've seen it work so many times.

Warning: never leave a suicidal person alone, even if this person wants to go to the bathroom. It is imperative to stand by and watch over them until help arrives.

An alternative to calling an ambulance and waiting for its arrival is to give the suicidal person the remedy and bring that person to the emergency room. Bottom line: A suicidal individual has to be brought to the hospital for professional observation.

And I'll say it again and again, and emphatically: NEVER LEAVE A SUICIDAL PERSON ALONE! STAY WITH THEM UNTIL PROFESSIONAL HELP ARRIVES OR THE PERSON IS BROUGHT SAFELY TO THE EMERGENCY ROOM!

Detoxification from Drugs, Alcohol, Nicotine, and Coffee

Detoxification is another area of human activities that calls for professional help. You've no doubt met some people who stopped smoking cigarettes on their own. Perhaps you've also met someone who stopped drinking on his or her own, and stayed sober for a long time. I knew one guy who stopped doing IV heroin on his own, and stayed away from it for at least a decade, which was as long as I knew him. Unfortunately, the majority of addicts cannot do it. They relapse. Even if they can stay away from an addictive substance for a while, the addiction comes right back when they're put under stress.

Rehabilitation centers and detoxification centers stay busy all the time. Promises of miraculous "rapid detox" in a few hours are many, but long-term results of such efforts are extremely poor. In my experience, homeopathy helps a drug or alcohol addict kick their habit for the long run if an experienced homeopath gets involved and that person also manages to stay sober for a few months during the initial treatment. The importance of peer support groups like Alcoholics Anonymous (AA), Narcotics Anonymous (NA), and similar organizations cannot be stressed enough.

Warning: Do not attempt to detoxify on your own if you are a habitual alcohol or drug abuser. Do not attempt discontinuation of alcohol or drugs "cold turkey," as it may lead to severe complications. Alcohol and drug withdrawal can lead to seizures and death in some cases. Seek professional medical help at the first signs of withdrawal: anxiety and/or tremors.

If you are addicted to street drugs, conventional medications (for example, painkillers), or alcohol, please seek conventional professional help. At this time dedicated homeopathic detoxification centers do not exist. Due to the importance of professional support, the suggestions for detoxification that follow apply only to the sporadic use of drugs, rather than habitual abuse, unless otherwise specified.

Before getting to the actual remedies, let me point out a side issue to the topic at hand. In our society, conventional prescription and over-the-counter medications are often overused, and even those that are properly used can produce adverse effects. The ultimate resolution of this problem is too complex to discuss in this short, narrowly focused book, however if you feel the need for treatment for potential side effects from taking conventional medications, homeopathy can frequently help. In some cases, homeopaths will prescribe homeopathic preparations derived from conventional medications that have caused complications. Certain types of treatment (for instance, cancer treatment) involve powerful immune suppressants. Some side effects of these pharmaceuticals can be treated with homeopathy.

Here are a few remedies that can help you or your family members to recover from the adverse effects of taking either street drugs or conventional medications.

Instructions: For temporary acute detoxification, take three pellets of your remedy of choice in 30C concentration daily until you see signs of significant improvement. Stop taking the remedy if no effect is noticeable in two to three days.

***Ignatia amara* (St. Ignatius' bean):** For overuse of street drugs or antidepressants and tranquilizers (these drugs are also frequently abused), when the individual:
- Feels a lump in their throat.
- Frequently yawns or sighs.
- Holds tears back and winds up sobbing.
- Has strange sensations in their body.

- Experiences numbness.
- Spasms and twitches.
- Experiences changeable symptoms, changeable moods.

***Avena sativa* (oats):** Many homeopaths report that *Avena sativa* is helpful for decreasing and stopping use of addictive substances, including marijuana, opiates (opium, heroin, morphine, cocaine), painkillers, tranquilizers, alcohol, coffee, and tobacco. Predictably, not everyone benefits from this remedy. Characteristic symptoms include:

- Severe exhaustion as a result of prolonged drug use, resulting in amenorrhea (lack of menstruation in young women), impotence, and poor concentration.
- Severe insomnia as a result of drug abuse.
- Headaches.

***Chamomilla* (German chamomile):** A major remedy for bad effects of coffee. Chief characteristics include:

- Sleeplessness until 2 AM.
- Irritability.
- Argumentativeness.
- Capriciousness.

***Ipecacuanha* (ipecac root):** For relief of severe nausea after chemotherapy. Look for signs, such as:

- **Constant nausea, which is not better after vomiting.**
- **Tongue is clean** despite stomach upset.
- Lack of thirst.
- The feeling of the stomach hanging loose.
- Possible abdominal cramps.

Nux vomica **(Quaker button):** This remedy is the best friend of drinkers with a morning hangover, as it reduces the symptoms. But remember: Any severe alcohol withdrawal after binge drinking (drinking large amounts, perhaps for an extended period of time) requires professional detoxification. In this case, take the remedy on your way to the ER.

Instructions: Take three pellets of 30C three to four times at fifteen-minute intervals, when you observe the following signs.

- Feeling burned out
- Irritability, anger, and argumentativeness
- Extreme sensitivity to light, odors, **noise,** and touch
- Urge to vomit or to pass a stool without any effect

Quercus glandium **(spirits of acorn):** This remedy helps to overcome alcohol cravings. It antidotes the negative effects of alcohol, such as:

- Depression with nervousness, tearfulness.
- Fear of a stroke.
- Vertigo.
- Noises in the head.
- Swollen abdomen due to enlarged liver and/or spleen.

Note: Diarrhea during treatment with *Quercus glandium* frequently signifies that the remedy is having a positive impact.

Insomnia

According to some estimates 14.5 percent of adult Americans suffer from insomnia.[6] That's one in seven. Regardless of how accurate this estimate is, we all know that many people have difficulties falling asleep and maintaining sleep. In my experience, professional constitutional treatment of insomnia can be successful if it is combined with better sleep hygiene and relaxation techniques. In new cases of insomnia, you also have to make sure that there are no serious underlying health problems.

Lack of sleep is not a trivial matter. We all know how difficult it is to go on if we don't get enough quality sleep each night. Yet treatment of insomnia is not easy. Insomnia is frequently a segment of a vicious cycle of a more serious disease. For example, a loss of sleep in someone's late teens or early twenties could be a sign of emerging bipolar disorder or clinical depression. Or it could be the result of an abnormally functioning thyroid gland. Or it could be the result of severe stress at work. Obviously I could go on and on.

When insomnia is a result of easily identified factors, a few herbal remedies, such as tea or extract made from hops or valerian root can be soothing. In my experience, supplementing with the hormone melatonin also provides significant relief for mild insomnia. If insomnia persists or it is already a chronic problem, you should have a thorough medical workup and consult an experienced homeopath for constitutional treatment.

Below, please find several homeopathic remedies that can be helpful in cases of simple, easy to understand insomnia. Anything beyond that really belongs in the realm of a trained homeopath. Ignatia is appropriate for treating insomnia that's the result of grief, a breakup, or bad news. Main characteristics to look for in cases of insomnia include:

- **Fear that the patient won't be able to fall asleep ever again.**
- Changeable moods.
- Wakes up crying.
- Frequent nervous yawning, sighing.
- Jerking of limbs on going to sleep.

Table 13.2 Insomnia Remedy Comparison Chart

Remedy	Reason for Insomnia
Arnica	Jet lag; recent accident
Calcarea phosphorica	Growth spurt (in children)
Chamomilla	Teething; colic; overuse of coffee; pain
China	Significant bleeding; prolonged breast-feeding; prolonged diarrhea; malaria
Cocculus	Night vigils (e.g., sitting up with a sick relative)
Coffea	Excitement
Gelsemium	Anticipation (like before a test or important presentation); flu; mononucleosis
Ignatia	Grief; bad news
Nux vomica	Abuse of alcohol, stimulants, or street drugs; overwork and stress; working too hard and playing too hard

SUPER REMEDIES | 315

Emotional State	Physical Symptoms and Modalities
Has vivid dreams or nightmares of an accident or injury	Extreme exhaustion with bruised feeling; bed feels hard
Discontented; constantly complaining	Shifting pains in the bones; exhaustion in the morning, even after a long sleep; tension in the neck and shoulders
Irritable; demanding; crying and moaning in sleep; child wants to be carried	Sleepy during the day but cannot sleep at night
Sensitive to noise; irritable; has many thoughts running through the head at night	Feeling of being very cold and weak
Worried about relatives or friends in need	Motion sickness; wakes up startled
Has high nervous energy; full of many thoughts and ideas	Very acute sense (to pain, touch, light, odors, sounds)
Mentally dull	Fall asleep in the early evening just to wake up in a few hours and not be able to go back to sleep; weakness with heaviness in the back of the head
Fearful of never falling asleep again; wakes up crying	Frequent nervous yawning and sighing; jerking of limbs on going to sleep
Irritable; angry; always on edge; irritated by noises	Wakes up around 3 AM full of thoughts about work and problems

Compare *Ignatia* to the following remedies.

Instructions: It is best to take one dose of any remedy you select in concentration 200C.

***Arnica montana* (leopard's bane):** For insomnia after a recent accident or jetlag. Main indicators of needing this remedy are:
- Nightmares or vivid dreams of an accident and injuries that the person had.
- Feeling extremely tired, but cannot sleep.
- Feeling bruised, with the bed feeling too hard.

***Calcarea phosphorica* (calcium phosphate):** For insomnia in children going through growth spurts or for insomnia after a long illness. *Instructions:* Take three to five tablets of a cell salt in potency 6X two to three times a day for a month. Major indicators are:
- Discontent and constant complaining. (Compare to *Chamomilla*.)
- Feeling tired in the morning even after a long sleep.
- Tension in the neck and shoulders.

***Chamomilla* (German chamomile):** Take for insomnia triggered by the overuse of coffee, drugs, and pain, or when a child cannot sleep due to teething and/or colic. Major characteristics are:
- Drowsiness during the day, sleeplessness at night.
- Irritability, capriciousness, being demanding.
- Child wants to be carried all the time.
- Crying and moaning in sleep.

***China (Chinchona officinalis)*:** For insomnia after loss of fluids, such as from bleeding, prolonged breast feeding, profuse sweating, or diarrhea. Signs of this remedy are:

- Many thoughts running in the head prevent a person from falling asleep.
- Extreme sensitivity (especially to noise).

Cocculus indicus **(Indian cockle):** The picture of this remedy includes:
- **Sleeplessness from exhaustion brought about by night vigils, like sitting up with a sick relative.**
- Waking up startled.
- Usually also has motion sickness.

Coffea cruda **(unroasted coffee):** The most frequently used homeopathic remedy for temporary relief of insomnia. *Note:* Do not be tempted to offer it to coffee drinkers, because *Chamomilla* is the right remedy for the abuse of caffeine. Use for:
- **Insomnia from excitement and too much enthusiasm.**
- A head that is full of ideas.
- Difficulty in falling asleep because of excitement and many thoughts.
- Extreme sensitivity to pain, touch, light, odors, and sounds.
- High nervous energy, even hyperactivity.

Gelsemium sempervirens **(yellow jasmine):** This remedy offers significant relief in cases of insomnia that are secondary to anticipation, overwork, over studying, and also to colds, the flu, mononucleosis, or a difficult pregnancy. Use it when you see:
- Head feels heavy, especially in the back.
- Mental dullness.
- Weakness.

- Falling asleep in the evening after supper, or watching TV, or studying. Wakes up an hour or two later and cannot go back to sleep.

Nux vomica **(Quaker button):** Often the remedy of choice for insomnia from anger, abuse of stimulants and drugs, and drinking too much alcohol or overeating the night before. It is also used for insomnia caused by overwork and stress—the typical modern businessperson's lifestyle. Look for signs like:
- Falling asleep early, then **waking up at 3 AM** full of thoughts about problems.
- Irritability, anger.
- Irritation from noises or any other interference.

Other Conditions That May Require *Ignatia*

As you may imagine, any condition with contradictory symptoms that develops in a person with a history of grief or significant loss could respond beautifully to *Ignatia*. A homeopath of my acquaintance, for example, couldn't figure out a remedy for one of her patient's mastitis (breast infection), and then found out the woman had lost a close and beloved relative a year earlier. After she gave her patient one dose of *Ignatia,* the mastitis disappeared. Now obviously, this homeopath was experienced and ran numerous possible solutions through her head before she restored to prescribing *Ignatia*. If she'd seen any symptoms of a more frequently used remedy for mastitis she would've tried that first.

When *Not* to Self-Medicate with *Ignatia*

Best to try a different remedy if you see:
- The person is in a severe depression. This condition requires professional help.
- Drug withdrawal.
- Alcohol withdrawal.
- Chronic insomnia.
- The picture of the remedy is unclear.

CHAPTER FOURTEEN

Nux Vomica Your Homeopathic Gastroenterologist

*"You don't get ulcers from what you eat.
You get them from what's eating you."*
—VICKI BAUM

Every homeopath in the world prescribes **Nux vomica (Quaker button, poison nut, *Strychnos nux-vomica*)** very frequently. The reason underlying such common use of this medication is simple: It is perfectly suited to the emotional and physical state triggered by the typical stressors of the modern lifestyle. Even in this short book, you've already "met" *Nux vomica* when potential remedies were being compared for insomnia, headaches, and drug detoxification. The individual who needs it feels stressed out and overworked.

Just for a moment, imagine an irritable businessman coming home late at night from work tired, hungry, and angry. Or imagine a woman who gets cranky for a few days before her period. Both individuals can feel their inner tension mounting by the minute. Although these images of those who benefit from *Nux vomica* are a bit like cartoons, when you consider taking this remedy or giving it to a member of your family, do please remember that people who need *Nux vomica* always possess at least a hint of anger and impatience. Combine these two important features with increased sensitivity to stimuli—sounds, light, and odors—and a *Nux vomica* picture truly emerges. Another highlight of this state of being is the presence of significant digestive problems. Those are its major indicators.

Although *Nux vomica* comes second to last in our list of seven important homeopathic remedies to keep on hand around your house, it is definitely not the least. In fact, one leading Indian homeopath, N.M. Choudhuri, calls it the "king of all remedies,"[1] as it can implement a cure for literally more than 10,000 symptoms. There is a term for exceptionally useful remedies like this one, of which there are only a handful.

"There are a few medicines, the majority of whose symptoms correspond in similarity with the symptoms of the commonest and most frequent of human diseases, and hence very often find an efficacious homoeopathic employment . . . They may be termed *polychrests,*" writes Samuel Hahnemann [my italics]. "To these belong particularly the nux vomica seed . . . it proves the mildest and most efficacious remedy in all the diseases whose symptoms correspond in similarity to the effects nux vomica is capable of producing in the healthy human being, when administered in the small doses."[2]

A polychrest is a homeopathic remedy that, because of its ability to heal many different mental, emotional, and physical ailments, has widespread use. Polychrest remedies have very prominent characteristics, so when you see any characteristics of a polychrest in a sick person, give it regardless of what specific ailment the person has.

In reality, a large proportion of our modern society often finds itself in the *Nux vomica* state—some due to their innate psychophysiological makeup, others driven to it by constant exposure to stimuli and pressure, which make them uncharacteristically irritable. Many of us can get over our symptoms just by resting, eating, and participating in relaxing activities. But some get stuck and need help from *Nux vomica,* the king.

The Origins of *Nux Vomica*

Nux vomica is a medium-sized tree native to India and Sri Lanka whose approximate height is twelve to fourteen meters. Its fruit, which is the size of a large apple, is filled with a jelly-like pulp and contains five seeds that are shaped like disks. One might compare these seeds to simple buttons, which is where the tree's folk name, Quaker button, originated. Because they are hard and therefore difficult to crush, the homeopathic remedy must be prepared starting from an alcohol extract of the "buttons."

As you learned in the previous chapter, *Ignatia amara* is the sister of *Nux vomica,* as these two remedies are made from closely botanically related plants. Like *Ignatia,* the chief constituents of *Nux vomica* are *strychnine* and *brucine,* which are contained in the tree and its fruit. However, while *Nux vomica* and *Ignatia* are akin and share two active ingredients, albeit in different proportions, their homeopathic actions are quite different.

Prominent American homeopath Robin Murphy writes: "The difference in the character of *Ignatia* and *Nux vomica* proves the wisdom of Hahnemann's simple methods of studying medicines. If there was nothing more than the chemistry of the drugs to go by Ignatia and Nux-v might be used indifferently [*for the same symptoms or illnesses—author*]. With the knowledge Hahnemann has given us of their characteristic features they are seldom even thought of in connection with the same case."[3] Indeed, as you'll soon see, *Nux vomica* is prescribed for people unlike those who need *Ignatia*.

Homeopathic provings have allowed us to perceive the fine distinctions between the qualities of various medicinal substances. Just to give you an idea of how significant the differences are in this particular case, let's investigate with the help of a computer. Modern homeopathic software offers many valuable features. The program RADAR, for example, enables us to analyze what symptoms are unique to one remedy in comparison with another. Accordingly, *Nux vomica* may cure 11,031 symptoms. *Ignatia*, only 5,988. In comparison to each other, out of all their catalogued symptoms, almost 70 percent of the symptoms of *Nux vomica* and 84 percent of the symptoms of *Ignatia* are particular to that remedy.

So, as you can clearly see, although these substances have produced some similar symptoms in provings (and thus could cure them), their dissimilarities are so significant that each remedy made from them corresponds to a distinguishable, well-defined state.

Indian folk medicine has found many applications for nonhomeopathic nux vomica. The bark is ground along with black pepper and then made into a paste that is given orally in a single dose for asthma attacks or labor pains. Interestingly, the same preparation is given three times a day for colds and coughs. The nux vomica seed is an ingredient in the Indian folk medicine for dog bites and in the external preparation for skin diseases. Leprosy is treated with the ground bark of the nux vomica tree.

Europeans first learned about this plant species from the German botanist Valerio Cordo who described it in 1561. Initially, products made from the tree were used to kill rodents and small predators. Fascinated by the poisonous power of the seeds, European scientists discovered that plants die after their roots are immersed in nux vomica extract. Subsequent studies showed that in small doses this plant could be helpful for various ailments. Only Hahnemann was able to discover the range of its medicinal applications.

Symptoms Characteristic of the *Nux Vomica* State

The attributes of the classic Type A personality closely match the description of typical symptoms calling for *Nux vomica*. According to Vijay P. Sharma, Ph.D., "There are two cardinal features of Type A that we must remember, namely, 'time urgency or time-impatience' and 'free-floating (all pervasive and ever-present) hostility.'"[4] Whereas Type B personalities are laid back and easygoing, Type A personalities are workaholics, always busy, driven, impatient, and so on. Likewise, someone in a *Nux vomica* state is impatient, angry, ambitious, and confident to the point of being arrogant.

Type A behavior was discovered and researched in the 1950s after two American cardiologists, Meyer Friedman, M.D., and Ray Rosenman, M.D., both noticed that the edges of chairs in their waiting rooms were worn out. They hypothesized that patients at high risk for coronary disease were driven, impatient people who impatiently sat on the edges of their seats before appointments. In 1974, they reported their insightful observations in a popular book, *Type A Behavior and Your Heart*.

Elaine Woo, a *New York Times* staff writer states: "'Type A personality' soon became part of the national vocabulary, shorthand for the sort of driven individual who feels oppressed by time. This is the person who honks and fumes in traffic, barks at sluggish salesclerks, and feels compelled to do several things at once—perhaps shave while paying bills and dialing a phone."[5]

Think about a person who requires *Nux vomica* as somebody who is born oversensitive, who therefore tenses up and strains too much. Any condition that begins with the following unique combination of symptoms can be improved by *Nux vomica*.

- Irritability due to an overall sensitivity to stimuli of all kinds
- Very easily offended
- Angry if contradicted
- Impatient
- Competitive
- Feels chilly
- Most symptoms are better from warmth, better in hot and humid weather
- Frequent digestive problems with spasmodic problems (for example, constipation with the main characteristic of urging for stool that does not resolve in passing the stool ("ineffectual urging").

While it is important to remember that some people are born to react in a "Nux vomica way," there are also some circumstances that may trigger this combination of symptoms, among them:

- Prolonged, stressful work.
- Working night shifts.
- Overindulgence in food and stimulants, such as coffee.
- Drug and alcohol abuse.

Digestive Problems

Before we delve into all the various remedies for digestive problems, I have an obligation to inform you honestly that our famous gastroenterologist, the King, has a rival. This polychrest, *Arsenicum album* (oxide of arsenic), is such a powerful contender that bestselling author Chris Bohjalian mentions the remedy several times in his novel *The Law of Similars*.[6] *Arsenicum album* is not included in our list of eight remedies for a simple reason. For acute ailments, perhaps with the exception of flu, colds, and diarrhea, its application is rarely obvious. Nonetheless this remedy remains important and you must be able to clearly understand the differences between it and *Nux vomica*.

The need for *Nux vomica* presents itself through symptoms that result from living life on overdrive. People in a *Nux vomica* state become increasingly sensitive and, as a result, irritable and cramped up. People who need *Arsenicum album* have a different set of issues. Usually they are suffering from a loss of structure or support, two things they need to feel OK in their lives. As a result, they feel anxious and restless, and ultimately become exhausted. Metaphorically speaking, while a "plant" person (*Nux vomica*) is sensitive, a "mineral" person (*Arsenicum*) thrives on structure. People who need *Nux vomica* are angry, whereas *Arsenicum* people are anxious. *Nux vomica* people tend to get constipated. *Arsenicum album* people tend to develop diarrhea.

People who need *Arsenicum album* have other unique characteristics, such as burning pains that get better from warm applications and heat, and a constant thirst for small sips of cold water. They also want fresh air. You might find a person who needs *Arsenicum album* bundled up with his head in close proximity to an open window.

Now let's compare *Nux vomica* with other remedies good for digestive problems.

Constipation

Nux vomica is one of the main remedies for constipation, especially spastic constipation. As this is frequently a complicated ailment to treat, perceiving a difference among the possible homeopathic remedies that might cure it requires professional training and years of experience. Use *Nux vomica* when you notice some of these characteristic symptoms.

- Constipation as a result of stressful, sedentary, overindulgent lifestyle
- Constipation associated with hemorrhoids (also see the section on page 342)
- Frequent desire for stool, but urging is ineffective
- Frequently goes to the bathroom, strains, but passes only small quantities
- **Feeling of unfinished, unsatisfactory stool**—keeps going back to achieve completion
- Constipation that alternates with diarrhea
- Irritability, with headaches and upset stomach

Here, I am listing only two other basic remedies with obvious, easy-to-appreciate symptoms, as I've seen so many cases in which one of these three remedies made a big difference. Try your best to match *Nux vomica* or one of these alternatives to your condition. Then take three to five pellets of your chosen remedy in 12C potency twice a day for a week or two. If your condition doesn't improve during that time period, seek the guidance of a trained homeopath. Some people may need to repeat their chosen remedy later, after an initial improvement, but this need typically will occur less and less often.

***Alumina* (aluminum):** This remedy is especially good for older people, during pregnancy, and for constipated newborns and bottle-fed infants. Watch for the following signs.

- No desire for stool. In infants, desire appears only when there is a large amount of stool. They may experience painful urging
- Pregnant women report a sensation of extreme dryness in the rectum
- It requires straining hard to pass even a soft stool. In some cases, the stool has to be removed by hand
- Stool is dry, hard, and comes out in knots
- Cutting pains in anus while passing stool, possible bleeding

The following symptoms don't necessarily have to be present, but if they are, then your remedy for sure should be *Alumina*.

- Mental dullness, confusion, slow to answer
- Aversion to potatoes or stomach easily gets upset by eating potatoes (I know it sounds strange; nonetheless, it is a valuable symptom)

***Bryonia alba* (white bryony):** Like *Alumina*, this remedy is quite helpful for elderly people and pregnant women. It is also useful in treating infants, especially when they're teething. Signs that it is the right remedy to take include:

- No desire for stool (similar to *Alumina*, yet the other indications are different)
- Stool is dry and **looks burned**
- Irritability (compare to *Nux vomica*)
- Headache that is made much worse by even the slightest movement

Table 14.1 Constipation Remedy Comparison Chart

Remedy	Better	Worse	Emotional state
Alumina	No specific modalities	Potatoes	Dull confused (gets clearer by the end of the day)
Bryonia	Rest	No specific modalities	Irritable
Nux vomica	Warmth; a complete bowel movement	Cold; emotional stress	Irritable; angry

- Constipation improves from rest
- Dry mouth with coated tongue
- Bad, bitter taste in the mouth
- Very thirsty for large amounts of cold liquids

Diarrhea

Once I consulted with a couple that shared the same main complaint: they got diarrhea when traveling to an Asian country. I'd previously seen them both for issues unrelated to digestion. From our earlier meetings, I recalled that the wife was an anxious person and the husband was a high-powered businessman. The original matters had resolved quickly. Easy

Physical Problems	Signs Guiding Your Selection	Food cravings
Vertigo on closing the eyes; dryness of the mouth, rectum, and skin	No urging for stool; constipation during pregnancy with extremely dry rectum; constipation with soft stool	Craving for dry foods (e.g., dry rice); craving for inedible things (e.g., earth, coal, chalk); aversion to potatoes
Bitter taste in the mouth; headache that is made much worse by even the slightest movement	No desire to pass a stool; burnt-looking stool	Craving for large amounts of cold liquids
Chill; generally worse in the morning	Strong urges to pass a stool but with very little output; feeling of needing to go again after a bowel movement	Craving for stimulants (e.g., coffee, alcohol, and spicy food)

come-easy go. As a homeopath, when a case was easy if you see the patient a year or two later you can't remember what remedy you prescribed without looking it up in your notes. A difficult case is a totally different story.

So they came in, and I began with the wife. The first comment out of her mouth was that she'd also made appointments with an infectious disease specialist and a holistic doctor known to checks for parasites, "just to make sure" that she hadn't contracted an incurable tropical illness. I offered her a glass of cool water and she sipped it frequently throughout the interview in small portions. She rearranged all the toys I keep for kids in my office. She complained that her stool was frequent and burning. If you are thinking about the remedy *Arsenicum album* at this point, you are correct. That's what I gave her.

When it was the husband's turn, he came in and I saw that he was irritated. He had just had a huge argument in the waiting room with another patient over who got to use the phone first (this happened a few years ago, when people were not as attached to their cell phones yet). He needed to make a few important phone calls. After the man calmed down, I gently pushed him into a conversation about competitive sports. It turned out that he played tennis and golf. He readily reported that he needed to win all the time and that if he lost he might lose not only the game but also his temper. His food desires were "very traditional." He drank coffee a few times a day, ate rich, spicy food, and had a few drinks after work. He also complained of waking up in the middle of the night thinking about business matters. Furthermore, his diarrhea was special. He had a lot of cramps and felt that his bowel movements, although liquid, were incomplete and unsatisfactory. The man received *Nux vomica* and he got excellent results.

Diarrhea is one of the few conditions for which the benefits of homeopathy have been repeatedly demonstrated in well-designed clinical studies. The leading researcher is Jennifer Jacobs, M.D., past president of the American Institute of Homeopathy. Here *Nux vomica*'s rival *Arsenicum* definitely has the upper hand, nonetheless, you would select *Nux vomica* if someone were to exhibit the following symptoms.

- **Frequent ineffectual urges** to have a bowel movement
- Cramping with painful diarrhea with the urge to go again soon after stool (feels incomplete)
- **Diarrhea after excessive use of alcohol**
- Diarrhea after experiencing stress related to work and business
- Diarrhea after anger
- Better from warm applications to the abdomen (compare to *Arsenicum*)

Among other things, through her research Jacobs learned that *Arsenicum* is one of the five most frequently prescribed homeopathic remedies for diarrhea in children.[7] These results hold true for adults, too. Nonetheless, you have many more excellent options from which to choose, at least eight of high merit. Consider this list.

Aloe **(aloes):** Signs to use this remedy include:
- Sudden urging for stool in the morning that literally drives a person out of bed (compare to *Sulphur*)
- Urge for stool at 5 AM (compare to *Sulphur*)
- **Diarrhea accompanied by a lot of gas and sputtering**
- Involuntary stool on passing gas
- Stool contains jelly-like parts of mucus
- Better from lying on the abdomen

Argentum nitricum **(silver nitrate):** Signs to use this remedy include:
- **Diarrhea from anxious anticipation, after mental or emotional strain.** (Compare to *Gelsemium*)
- Diarrhea is accompanied with abdominal rumbling, bloating, and gas (an important point to distinguish from the symptoms of *Gelsemium*)
- A person feels very warm
- The person is extroverted, cheerful, perhaps too open, and cocky. (Compare this to the shy, quiet type who benefits from *Gelsemium*)
- Worse immediately after drinking water and from lying on the left side, sweets (that someone usually craves), and heat
- Better from burping, which can be pretty loud

Table 14.2 Diarrhea Remedy Comparison Chart

Remedy	Better	Worse	Emotional State	Physical Problems
Aloe	Lying on abdomen	Overeating; beer; oysters; unripe fruit; 5 to 6 AM	No specific symptoms for this condition	Feels warm; dislikes heat
Argentum nitricum	Burping (can be loud)	Drinking; ice cream; sweets; heat	Warm; extroverted; a bit too open; cocky; lovable; morbidly afraid of heights	Feels hot and bloated
Arsenicum	Heat; warm applications (e.g., hot water bottle) to the abdomen	Cold environment; cold food and drink; fruit; meat; alcohol; between midnight and 2 AM	Anxious; antsy; detail oriented	Always cold; irritating, burning stool; often has significant nausea and vomiting
Chamomilla	Being constantly carried	Heat; being angry; night	Irritable; demanding; capricious	Green stool that looks like spinach or chopped grass and has the odor of rotten eggs

Signs Guiding Your Selection	Food Cravings and Aversions	Remedy to Compare With
Sudden urge for stool in the morning; lots of gas; involuntary stool on passing gas	Craving for juicy things; aversion to meat	*Arsenicum; Podophyllum; Sulphur*
Diarrhea from anxious anticipation (stage fright)	Craving for sweets	*Gelsemium; Sulphur*
Food poisoning; overeating fruit; diarrhea every morning in the elderly; chronic diarrhea in alcoholics	Craving for water in small sips; craving for sour things, whiskey, wine, and fat (also likes warm food)	*Argentum nitricum; Gelsemium; Veratrum album*
Diarrhea in infants and small children; diarrhea during teething and colic	Craving for coffee (in adults)	*Nux vomica; Sulphur*

Table 14.1 Diarrhea Remedy Comparison Chart *(continued)*

Remedy	Better	Worse	Emotional State	Physical Problems
China	Warmth; plenty of liquids	Nursing (for babies); significant loss of blood or other bodily fluids; fruit, fish, and milk; every other day, or any other periodicity; night	Sensitive to all stimuli; has many thoughts running in the head; may be apathetic	Feels very cold; significant indigestion (feels like food is just lying in the stomach); very weak; pale with large circles under the eyes
Gelsemium	No specific modalities for this problem	Anticipation; thinking about illnesses; walking	Timid; anxious; likes to be alone	Trembling from anxiety; fatigued; sticky sweat all over body
Nux vomica	Warmth; a complete bowel movement	Cold, emotional stress	Irritable; angry	Chilly; generally feels worse in the morning
Podophyllum	Cramps are better from passing stool (temporarily)	Hot weather; eating or drinking; early morning (4 to 5 AM)	Not much going on emotionally	Weak; feels like fainting; empty sensation in the stomach after passing a stool

Signs Guiding Your Selection	Food Cravings and Aversions	Remedy to Compare With
Diarrhea after prolonged exhausting diseases and after blood loss; hungry without appetite	Craves sour fruit	*Arsenicum; Gelsemium*
Diarrhea from anticipation	No thirst	*Argentum nitricum; Arsenicum*
Strong urges for stool but with very little output	Craving for stimulants (coffee, alcohol, spicy food)	
Severe diarrhea when stool is explosive and soils the entire toilet bowl and even the buttocks	No specific cravings or aversions	*Arsenicum; Sulphur*

Table 14.1 Diarrhea Remedy Comparison Chart *(continued)*

Remedy	Better	Worse	Emotional State	Physical Problems
Sulphur	No modalities specific for this condition	Beer; sweets; milk; early morning (5 to 6 AM)	Warm and open; can be short-tempered but quickly calms down; remains cheerful and in good spirits	Feels hot; stool burns and smells very bad
Veratrum album	Warmth	Extreme heat or cold	Often described as "sullen indifference"; feels wasted	Exhaustion; cold sweat, especially on forehead

***Arsenicum album* (oxide of arsenic):** Consider using this remedy first in cases of food poisoning. Other signs to use it are:

- Diarrhea may be accompanied by nausea and vomiting (compare to *Veratrum*)
- Chronic diarrhea in alcoholics
- Morning diarrhea in the elderly
- Stool is liquid, frequently looks like rice water, caustic, and **burning**
- The person is thirsty for small sips of cold water
- Chilly, anxious, restless
- May feel a fear of dying from diarrhea or some terrible underlying illness
- Worse between midnight and 2 AM
- Better from the application of warmth to the abdomen

Signs Guiding Your Selection	Food Cravings and Aversions	Remedy to Compare With
Offensive, burning diarrhea	Craving for cold drinks; craving for sweets, carbs, and spicy food; aversion to fish (although there are exceptions to this rule)	*Podophyllum*
Simultaneous diarrhea and projectile vomiting; exhaustion; excessive cold sweat	Craving for ice-cold drinks, as well as for salty and sour food	*Arsenicum*

Chamomilla **(German chamomile):** Often appropriate for treating diarrhea in infants and toddlers, especially when symptoms emerge in combination with teething.

- Sensitive, irritable, complaining
- **Capricious (asks for things that are later rejected)**
- **Wants to be carried all the time**
- Stool is green, has the odor of rotten eggs (compare with *Sulphur*)

China **(*Chinchona officinalis,* Peruvian bark):**

- Diarrhea during or after prolonged, exhausting illnesses (for example, AIDS) or following the loss of fluids, such as results from heavy bleeding or prolonged nursing

- **Diarrhea only at night**
- Tremendous weakness, sometimes with trembling
- Wants sour fruit, but develops diarrhea after eating fruit
- Pale with dark circles under the eyes

Gelsemium sempervirens (yellow jasmine):
- **Diarrhea from anticipation or fright** (compare to *Argentum*)
- Diarrhea is painless
- Diarrhea can be accompanied by frequent urination
- The person is weak and shy

***Podophyllum* (May apple):** This remedy is a specialist for the treatment of diarrhea. A famous homeopath Roger Morrison writes: "The efficacy of *Podophyllum* in acute diarrhea is so marked that our thoughts turn automatically to this remedy in such a condition, and must be forced by symptoms to look elsewhere."[8]

To make the differentiation between this remedy and *Arsenicum* crystal clear, the rule of thumb is always to consider this remedy first in cases of severe diarrhea, and think first of *Arsenicum* in cases of food poisoning. Other remedies are only prescribed when you can see their most prominent symptoms, or if you cannot find clear symptoms of either *Podophyllum* or *Arsenicum*.

People who need *Podophyllum* do not show a lot of anxiety; they are simply tired and exhausted from having diarrhea. Look also for:
- **Abundant, watery, noisy, explosive diarrhea.**
- Much gas.
- Stool soils the entire toilet bowl and the buttocks.
- Worse from heat, hot weather, in the morning around 4 AM to 5 AM (compare to *Arsenicum)*, and any motion.
- **Feels like fainting, very weak.**
- Gurgling before stool.

- Empty sensation after stool.
- Stool often has terrible offensive odor.
- May have a headache from diarrhea.
- Possible rectal prolapse from diarrhea.

Sulphur **(brimstone):** Signs to use this remedy include:
- **Urgent stool wakes the person around 5 AM and 6 AM** (compare to *Podophyllum*).
- Stool is painful with soreness and burning of anus.
- Stool has a horrific odor, frequently described as similar to the odor of rotten eggs. The entire household knows that the person is having a bowel movement, and people cannot enter the bathroom for a long time the smell is so foul.
- Feels hot during diarrhea (*Arsenicum* is for a person who feels a chill).
- Frequently remains hungry and cheerful.
- May fall asleep immediately after the fit of diarrhea.
- Thirsty for large amounts of cold drinks.

Veratrum album **(white hellebore):** Use this remedy if you see the following signs.
- **The key to this remedy is severe exhaustion,** which accompanies symptoms that look like *Arsenicum* symptoms, but without any anxiety
- **Diarrhea accompanied by cold sweats, especially on the forehead**
- **Diarrhea simultaneously with profuse forceful vomiting** (compare to *Arsenicum*)
- The person is exhausted, weak, and may even faint after stool
- Sometime a person reports a peculiar sensation of feeling coldness in the abdomen
- Worse from heat (compare to *Arsenicum*)

Hemorrhoids

Treatment of this problem can be complicated, particularly in cases where hemorrhoids are merely a segment of a complex set of health issues. That said, even the external use of homeopathic preparations can provide significant relief. In fact, most hemorrhoid sufferers whom I've seen in my practice swear by suppositories and ointments. You can easily locate these types of products in health food stores that carry homeopathic preparations. All of the major homeopathic companies make them.

Please be mindful of two important points before you start on a course of self-treatment for hemorrhoids.

1. Consult with your primary physician to find out as much as you can about the underlying cause of your hemorrhoids.
2. If you are under the care of a homeopath for any reason, please do not self-prescribe for hemorrhoids, especially if your main complaint has been improving. Give the remedy you're taking, or have taken, a chance to produce a cure.

Nux vomica is appropriate for extremely sensitive, painful hemorrhoids that appear in combination with stubborn constipation. It is appropriate when you see several items from the following constellation of symptoms.

- Hemorrhoids after overindulgence (too much coffee, too much alcohol)
- Hemorrhoids after abuse of laxatives
- Irritability, being on edge
- Worse from alcohol, stimulants, and motion
- Better after stool

Now let's talk about several additional remedies. These are the ones I find most frequently indicated and they are easy to distinguish. If you find choosing the correct remedy from the short list provided below too difficult in your case or the case of your family member, or if you would like to enhance the action of your current homeopathic or allopathic treatment for this condition, remember what you learned a few paragraphs ago about using homeopathic ointments or suppositories to gain temporary relief.

Aesculus **(horse chestnut):** This is the core remedy in most homeopathic ointments and suppositories for hemorrhoids. It is also correct to take it in tablet form when:
- **Painful hemorrhoids are associated with lower back pain.**
- **There's a feeling that the rectum is filled with splinters.**
- There's a sensation that the stool is rough or coarse.
- Hemorrhoids occur during pregnancy.
- Worse from standing.
- Better in a kneeling position and from taking a warm bath.

Aloe **(aloes):** This remedy is useful when:
- **Large hemorrhoids protrude like a bunch of grapes.**
- There's a loose or uncomfortably open, dragging sensation in rectum.
- In some cases, release of the stool is involuntary, especially on passing gas.
- Worse from sitting, during menses.
- Better from **cold bathing** (compare to *Sulphur*).

Table 14.3 Hemorrhoids Remedy Comparison Chart

Remedy	Better	Worse	Emotional State	Physical Problems
Aesculus	Kneeling; warm bath	Standing	Irritable	Lower back weakness and pain; feeling as if rectum is filled with splinters; hemorrhoidal pains that last hours after passing stools
Aloe	Cold bath	Sitting; beer	No specific symptoms for this condition	Loose feeling in the rectum, as if the sphincter is wide open; burning from passing gas; involuntary stool
Hamamelis	No specific modalities	Warmth and heat	No specific symptoms for this condition	Raw, sore anus
Ignatia	Walking or sitting (paradoxical modalities)	Emotional upset; passing a stool; lying down at night (paradoxical modalities)	Easily hurt; hysterical; touchy and defensive	Paradoxical reactions; feels better in the rain but worse from lying down, and so on; back spasms from grief; lump in the throat (could be in the rectum)

Signs Guiding Your Selection	Food Cravings and Aversions	Remedy to Compare With
Painful hemorrhoids plus lower back pain; hemorrhoids during pregnancy	No specific cravings or aversions for this problem	*Nux vomica; Paeonia; Ratanhia*
Large hemorrhoids protruding like a bunch of grapes	Craving for juicy things; aversion to meat	*Hamamelis; Sulphur*
Large blue hemorrhoids that bleed easily	No specific data	*Aloe*
Hemorrhoids and fissures with extremely painful rectal spasms, as if a knife were stuck in the rectum; pain worse from emotional problems and better from walking and sitting	Craving for cheese; aversion to fruit	*Nux vomica; Ratanhia*

Table 14.3 Hemorrhoids Remedy Comparison Chart *(continued)*

Remedy	Better	Worse	Emotional State	Physical Problems
Nux vomica	Bowel movement	Alcohol; abuse of laxatives; any type of overindulgence; motion	Irritable; angry	Chilly; generally worse in the morning
Paeonia	Lying down after passing a stool with legs and buttocks held spread apart	Slightest touch; even wiping gently after a bowel movement	Can be nervous and anxious with bad dreams, even nightmares	May have ulcers on the skin
Ratanhia	Warm bath, lying down; walking slowly	Passing a stool	Obsessive thoughts with compulsive rituals	Tendency to have fissures in various locations of the body
Sulphur	Cold bath	Standing; beer; night in bed	Warm and open; can be short-tempered but quickly calms down; remains cheerful and in good spirits	Feels hot; burning stool that smells very bad; itchy rectum;, which gets worse from scratching

Signs Guiding Your Selection	Food Cravings and Aversions	Remedy to Compare With
Painful hemorrhoids plus lower back pain; hemorrhoids during pregnancy	Craving for stimulants (coffee, alcohol, and spicy food)	*Nux vomica;* *Ratanhia*
Extremely painful hemorrhoids after passing a stool (better from lying down with legs and buttocks held spread apart)	No specific data	*Aesculus;* *Ignatia;* *Nux vomica;* *Ratanhia*
Pain that gives the sensation of having broken glass in the rectum; combination of hemorrhoids and obsessive behavior	No specific data	*Ignatia;* *Nux vomica;* *Paeonia*
Large hemorrhoids with terrible itching	Craving for cold drinks; craving for sweets, cards, and spicy food; aversion to fish (although there are exceptions to this rule)	*Aesculus*

Hamamelis **(witch hazel):** Together with *Aesculus,* this remedy is frequently a component of hemorrhoid suppositories and ointments. Look for:
- Weakness of all veins, **varicose veins.**
- **Large, blue, protruding hemorrhoids that bleed during stool.**

Ignatia amara **(St. Ignatius' bean):** Look for:
- **Hemorrhoids with extremely painful rectal spasms that appear or get worse after emotional distress.**
- Pain feels like a metal rod or a knife was stuck in the rectum.
- Worse **from lying down at night,** emotional trouble, and at the end of stool (a paradoxical symptom. (compare to *Nux vomica* and *Ratanhia).*
- Better **from walking or sitting** (here we go again, a paradoxical symptom)

Paeonia **(peony):** Look for:
- Tremendous pain after stool (compare to *Ratanhia).*
- Worse from even the slightest touch while wiping after a bowel movement.
- Better **from lying with legs and buttocks spread.** (If clear, this symptom alone dictates the use of this remedy. If it's absent, think about *Ratanhia* instead).

Ratanhia **(mapato):** Look for:
- **Incredible, excruciating pain after stool.** May last for minutes, even hours.
- Many describe a sensation of having **broken glass** in the rectum.
- Worse **after stool** and from hard stool.
- Better from walking slowly, lying down, and taking a warm bath.

***Sulphur* (brimstone):** Look for:
- Hemorrhoids with **overpowering, irresistible itching.**
- A personality that is usually personable, extroverted, friendly, and emotionally warm, but poorly groomed.
- Warm-blooded.
- Stool is extremely malodorous.
- Worse at night (especially the itching), and from drinking beer or standing.
- Better from taking a cold bath.

Nausea and Vomiting

This section will cover a handful of remedies that resolve most cases of uncomplicated nausea and vomiting. Everyone knows how common both these problems are. Many people suffer from seasickness or carsickness. Pregnant women often complain about morning sickness. Other people get nauseous from overeating. And still others from food poisoning. Sadly, nausea is also frequently a complication of chemotherapy for cancer.

Please remember that persistent feelings of nausea and/or frequent vomiting need to be investigated by a physician. This caution is especially applicable to newborns, babies, and pregnant women. There are numerous easily treatable and potentially life-threatening causes of nausea and vomiting. Some are: alcohol abuse, drug abuse, premenstrual syndrome (PMS), pregnancy, food intolerance, peptic ulcer, vertigo, headache, hepatitis, and cancer. Don't hesitate long in seeking professional help if these problems are persistent, or if the initial nausea or vomiting is severe, or even if they were relieved by homeopathy. You should always consult with a trained homeopath when confronting serious and chronic problems, or if your initial attempts to find a correct remedy on your own have failed.

As you may be aware, many people have used raw slices of ginger, boiled ginger water, and ginger tea to decrease and even eliminate their feelings of nausea. Some also find it helpful to drink diluted apple cider vinegar. To prepare the latter concoction: combine one or two teaspoons of apple cider vinegar with a glass of cold water (or if you like it better, water at room temperature). You may also add honey to taste. Drink small sips of this beverage throughout the day.

The best tactic for overcoming nausea and vomiting with homeopathic remedies is to take three pellets of 30C concentration of a remedy after each episode of vomiting. If the remedy works, the episodes should become less frequent and disappear in the course of a day or two. For cases of nausea that arise during chemotherapy, take your chosen remedy once daily for the duration of chemotherapy and/or nausea.

Nux vomica may be appropriate for symptoms of nausea and vomiting that occur as a result of alcohol and drug abuse, for nausea during constipation, and for nausea accompanied by unsuccessful and painful attempts to vomit, cramps, and/or painful episodes of vomiting. Look also for characteristic signs, such as:

- **Anger, irritability.**
- **Hypersensitivity to stimuli: sounds, light, odors, touch, and so on.**
- Worse in the morning and from eating, alcohol, being angry, cold drinks.
- Better from lying down, warm drinks, and food.

If symptoms pertaining to *Nux vomica* are not present in your situation, try one of the following homeopathic remedies instead.

Aethusa cynapium (fool's parsley): Look for:
- **Vomiting in nursing babies.**
- **Vomits milk in curds.**
- A baby that becomes sleepy after vomiting, then hungry, then eats, then vomits.
- **Worse from milk.**

Arsenicum album (oxide of arsenic): Look for:
- **Food poisoning.**
- Burning pains in the stomach or along the esophagus that accompany vomiting.
- Anxious, fearful, and restless during vomiting or with nausea.
- Feeling chilly.
- Vomiting accompanied by diarrhea. (Compare with *Veratrum album.*)
- Thirsty for sips of cold drinks, but vomits immediately after drinking them. (Compare to *Phosphorus.*)
- Worse after midnight, from cold drinks, and from the smell or even the thought of food. (If this last symptom is intense, compare with *Colchicum.*)
- Better from warm liquids.

Antimonium crudum (antimony sulphide): Look for:
- **Tongue that has a thick, white coat.**
- You cannot see any typical symptoms of other remedies.
- Worse from drinking, becoming warm, rich foods, and wheat-containing foods.

Bryonia alba (white bryony): Look for:
- **Vomiting provoked by even a slightest motion.**

- Worse from motion, trying to sit up in bed, raising the head, coughing.
- Better **from lying still, cold drinks** (compare to *Arsenicum album*).

Cocculus indicus **(Indian cockle):** Use when there is:
- **Motion sickness.** (Always compare to *Tabacum*. *Cocculus* is worse from open air, *Tabacum* is better from open air).
- **Nauseous when watching moving objects.** (Nausea in people who need this remedy comes from the brain, not from the stomach).
- Nausea in people exhausted by night vigilance (for example, sitting up with a severely ill friend or relative).
- Extreme weakness, even to the point of trembling.
- A person cannot tolerate the smell of food or even think of food. (Compare to Arsenicum and *Colchicum*.)
- Worse from motion.
- Better from lying on a side or being in a warm room. (Compare to *Tabacum*.)

Colchicum **(meadow saffron):** Use when:
- **Nauseous from the odor, sight, or even the thought of food.**
- Feeling faint from exposure to food odors. (**Often required by pregnant women with this particular symptom.**)
- Highly sensitive to rudeness.

Ipecacuanha **(ipecac root):** Signs to use this remedy include:
- **Awful nausea not at all relieved by vomiting.** (Compare to *Sanguinaria*.)

- Despite digestive problems and nausea, the tongue remains red and clean. (Compare to *Antimonium.*)
- Better except for this remedy, nothing makes this nausea feel better.

In my experience, it's often helpful for nausea during or after chemotherapy.

Kreosotum **(beachwood creosote):** Look for symptoms like:
- Nausea and **vomiting up of food undigested long after eating**
- Drinking water produces bitter taste.
- Vomiting occurs during PMS or pregnancy.
- Worse before menses and during pregnancy, and from cold food and meat.

Phosphorus **(phosphorus):** Signs include:
- **Vomiting from imbibing cold drinks, after they become warm in the stomach** (not immediately like in *Arsenicum*).
- Craving large amounts of cold drinks (compare to *Arsenicum's* small sips).
- Often remains cheerful and functions OK despite vomiting. (Compare to *Arsenicum* and *Veratrum.*)
- Worse from warm drinks and food (compare to *Nux vomica*), and **after general anesthesia** (a remedy of choice for this problem).
- Better temporarily from cold drinks, **after sleep**, and from lying on the right side.

Table 14.4 Nausea and Vomiting Remedy Comparison Chart

Remedy	Better	Worse	Emotional State	Physical Problems
Aethusa	Company; open air	Heat; summer; evening	Irritable; tearfulness	Gets colicky, irritable, and exhausted and then goes to sleep
Antimonium crudum	Open air; rest	Drinking; becoming warm; carbs	Difficult to please, irritable, contradictive; children don't like to be touched or looked at; adults are less obvious about those things	Thick, white-coated tongue; dry lips
Arsenicum	Warm drinks	Cold drinks; the smell and even the thought of food; midnight	Anxious; fearful (afraid of having a serious illness)	Cold, burning pains in the stomach with every fit of vomiting; vomiting may be accompanied by diarrhea
Bryonia	Lying absolutely still; being left alone; cold drinks	Even the slightest movement	Irritable	Dry, dirty-looking tongue

Signs Guiding Your Selection	Food Cravings and Aversions	Remedy to Compare With
Vomiting curds of milk soon after nursing	Little baby—eats only mother's milk or formula	
Nausea with indigestion; tongue covered with thick white coating	Craving for sour food, including pickles	*Bryonia; Ipecacuanha; Nux vomica*
Food poisoning; vomiting of cold drinks immediately after swallowing	Craving for sips for cold water	*Colchicum; Phosphorus; Veratrum*
Nausea provoked by the slightest movement	Craving for large amounts of cold water	*Veratrum*

Table 14.4 Nausea and Vomiting Remedy Comparison Chart *(continued)*

Remedy	Better	Worse	Emotional State	Physical Problems
Cocculus	Lying on the left side; warm room	Movement or even watching objects move; open, cold air	Full of concerns; may be irritable	Vertigo; metallic taste
Colchicum	Leaning forward	Odor, sight, or even thought of food; pregnancy	No relevant data	Extremely weak; feels cold inside or has burning and distension of the stomach; pupils may be of different size (confirms the remedy but is not always present)
Ipecacuanha	Nothing makes nausea better except for this remedy	Periodically, lying down	May be irritable	Clean, red tongue despite nausea
Kreosotum	Warmth; warm food	Time before menses and during pregnancy; cold food	Capricious	Vomits several hours after eating; has bitter taste upon swallowing water

Signs Guiding Your Selection	Food Cravings and Aversions	Remedy to Compare With
Motion sickness	Craving for cold drinks, especially beer; complete aversion to any type of food	*Kreosotum; Tabacum*
Nausea and vomiting of pregnancy	Craving for many types of food (but nauseous at the sight of them); craving for alcohol	*Arsenicum; Kreosotum; Sepia*
Severe nausea with no relief, even from vomiting	No specific data	*Antimonium*
Vomiting several hours after eating; nausea before menses and during pregnancy	No specific data	*Sepia*

Table 14.4 Nausea and Vomiting Remedy Comparison Chart *(continued)*

Remedy	Better	Worse	Emotional State	Physical Problems
Nux vomica	Lying down; warm drinks and food	Being angry; cold drinks and food; morning	Irritable; oversensitive; angry	Chilly; constipated
Phosphorus	Lying on the right side; sleep	Warm drinks and food; general anesthesia	Cheerful	Remains in good shape despite nausea and vomiting
Sanguinaria	Vomiting; acidic food; sleep; darkness	Sweets; motion	No specific data	Various right-sided problems (e.g., migraine)
Sepia	Eating; strenuous exercise	Time before breakfast	Cries easily; may be depressed; decreased energy from 3 to 5 PM	Exhausted; most complaints are better from exercise
Tabacum	Open, fresh air (like on the deck of a moving ship or by the open window of a moving car)	Extreme heat or cold	May be irritable	Extremely pale coloring (described by some as green)

Signs Guiding Your Selection	Food Cravings and Aversions	Remedy to Compare With
Nausea and vomiting from drug and alcohol abuse and constipation; cramps in the stomach during vomiting	Craving for stimulants (alcohol and rich, spicy food)	*Arsenicum*
Vomiting of cold drinks after they become warm in the stomach	Craving for cold water and salty things	*Arsenicum; Nux vomica; Veratrum*
Nausea and all other complaints much better after vomiting; nausea with salivation	Unquenchable thirst; aversion to butter	
Morning sickness of pregnancy; nausea after chemotherapy	Sour, sweet and sour food	*Colchicum; Kreosotum; Ipecacuanha*
Severe nausea (usually seasickness or car sickness) better from fresh air	No specific data (though some people crave tobacco)	*Cocculus*

Table 14.4 Nausea and Vomiting Remedy Comparison Chart *(continued)*

Remedy	Better	Worse	Emotional State	Physical Problems
Veratrum album	Night after sleep	Walking; warmth	In a stupor from exhaustion	Exhausted with cold sweat on the forehead and cold breath

Sanguinaria canadensis **(blood root):** Use when:
- **All symptoms are greatly relieved by vomiting.**
- **Migraines are right-sided.**
- Vomitus is bitter, caustic.

Sepia **(cuttle fish ink):** One of the most important remedies for morning sickness in pregnancy, *Sepia* is also an important potential remedy for nausea after chemotherapy. (Compare to *Ipecacuanha*.) Characteristic symptoms include:
- Motion sickness.
- In cases of morning sickness, a woman cannot tolerate her partner's smell.
- A woman feels weak and indifferent to people she usually loves.
- May have post-nasal discharge.
- Worse before breakfast, during sex, or even from a thought of sex.
- Better from eating (especially sour food) and from strenuous exercise.

Tabacum **(tobacco):** Consider for the following symptoms.
- **Very important for cases of seasickness** (amazingly, in days of yore most of the pirates and old skippers smoked a pipe)
- Deathly, severe nausea

Signs Guiding Your Selection	Food Cravings and Aversions	Remedy to Compare With
Projectile vomiting simultaneously with diarrhea	Craving for ice-cold water and salty things (even raw salt)	*Arsenicum; Phosphorus*

- **The person becomes extremely pale**, some people describe the color as "green"
- **Lightheadedness with cold sweat, a feeling one is about to faint**
- Better **from open air** (compare with *Cocculus*)

Veratrum album **(white hellebore):** The picture of this remedy includes the following symptoms.
- **Projectile vomiting simultaneously with diarrhea**
- **Complete exhaustion with cold sweat on the forehead, and sometimes cold breath**
- Often craves ice-cold drinks and/or ice, and craves salt
- Worse after sleep (compare with *Phosphorus*)

Hay Fever and Other Acute Allergies

In addition to being a gastroenterologist, *Nux vomica* has another terrific specialty. It's an allergist. As I mentioned before, polychrests like *Nux vomica* can be used to treat many different conditions with thousands of symptoms. Long live the King!

Seasonal allergies (aka hay fever) are enormously common, affecting at least 35.9 million people in the United States alone. In fact, approximately 16.7 million office visits to U.S. health care providers each year are attributed to allergic rhinitis. The American Academy of Allergy Asthma and Immunology offers these additional statistics:[9]

- Allergic diseases affect more than 20 percent of the U.S. population.
- Estimates from a skin test survey suggest that allergies affect as many as 40 to 50 million people in the United States.
- Allergic diseases are the sixth leading cause of chronic disease in the United States.

Interestingly, homeopaths pioneered both the research and the treatment of allergies. In 1871, British homeopath Charles H. Blackley suggested that seasonal sneezing and nasal discharge were the result of exposure to pollen. Later, James Tyler Kent defined the practical principles of treating allergies with homeopathy. If someone develops an acute reaction to pollen (or another allergen), such as a running nose or itching, watery eyes, during the allergy season, this reaction is addressed first. After all, there is no need for anyone to suffer discomfort. Then, during the symptom-free season, a homeopath aims to find a so-called constitutional remedy that solves the problem on every level of a person's being. It can take a while for the full effects of a remedy like this to be felt. But in the end, many other complaints usually drop away along with the symptoms of allergy.

Today conventional allergists use a desensitization process that resembles the homeopathic practice of "using like to cure like." They give their patients a bit of the allergen to stimulate a reaction that the body overcomes, thus making the body stronger. However, their injections do not feature homeopathically prepared solutions. It's a little known fact that a homeopath, Grant L. Selfridge, M.D., was the first president of the organization that is now the American Academy of Allergy, Asthma, and Immunology.

Here is an interesting educational case from my practice. As often happens, a family member who was cured from a longstanding migraine headache asked me whether I could help a man with severe seasonal allergies. Because it was allergy season, I saw a window of opportunity to come in with a homeopathic remedy at a time when all his shields were down—to address his raw, painful symptoms. The man came in the next week and presented, as his main complaint, frequent sneezing. Sometimes he sneezed more than ten times in a row right on waking up. The remedy listed in this chapter for this symptom is *Sabadilla*. Everyone who knows homeopathy will tell you that with this symptom alone the likelihood of the patient needing *Sabadilla* is high.

The next step in my thinking process (and it should also be the next step in yours) was to see what other characteristic mental symptoms, generalities, and modalities I could find. If there were no mental symptoms and the patient had told me that the only other symptoms he had were sneezing (mostly in the morning) and having his palate itch, *Sabadilla* would move right to the top of the list possible remedies and win. But the man also complained of waking up every night around 3 am thinking about his new job.

In addition, he said that his nose felt stuffed all the time. He was pretty intense, on the edge, irritable, and easily offended. He said he needed to eat a lot of dark chocolate every day (in my head this is a stimulant similar to coffee). He also said that even though he knew that spices make his sneezing worse, he ate Indian food almost every day. He complained of constipation and told me that after he sneezed, he felt unsatisfied, like he needed to sneeze more to finish the job. Using your imagination, can you easily imagine that this feeling of incompleteness after a sneeze is not so different from the feeling of incompleteness after a bowel movement? In the big picture, that is.

Guess what? I gave him *Nux vomica*. It was total success. As you can see very clearly from this case, I just went with the flow of his symptoms. I did not pull anything out of him with forceps. It was a clean, simple case with an easy (for you and I) solution. You'll probably see more cases of *Sabadilla, Euphrasia,* and *Allium cepa* (all described below) for hay fever, but remember that *Nux vomica* is always standing by, just in case.

This book offers you a few solutions for simple acute problems, such as might arise during allergy season, or after eating an unfamiliar food. Beside the homeopathic remedies, I also recommend trying a combination of one or more of the following natural solutions, as these are often very effective.

1. *Extract of eyebright and stinging nettles.* (Herb Pharm has a product called Eyebright/Nettle Compound and other herbal companies have similar products). *Dose:* Take ten drops three times a day. As you read forward, you'll notice that homeopathic preparations of both of these herbs are listed for the treatment of allergies. Don't worry about taking the herbs and remedies simultaneously. Nonhomeopathic preparations of herbs do not counteract the effects of homeopathy.
2. *Bioflavonoids.* I recommend taking between 3,000 and 4,000 milligrams a day (each tablet or capsule contains 1,000 mg).
3. *Eliminate wheat and/or dairy from your diet.* For some people, eliminating wheat and dairy does miracles. For others, it has no impact on their allergies.

Nux vomica is the correct remedy for your own or your family's allergies if you see the following characteristic symptoms.

- Sneezing and discharge from the nose upon **rising from bed in the morning**
- **Dry, sore, stuffed nose at night while in bed**

- Irritability
- Worse on waking up in the morning, after meals, and from open air
- Better from being in a **warm room** (in some cases, the nose completely clears up) and from warm drinks

If those symptoms are not present, consider one of the following remedies instead.

Allium cepa **(red onion):** Always compare to *Euphrasia*.
- **Irritating, caustic discharge from the nose that irritates the nose and the upper lip** (opposite of *Euphrasia*)
- **Bland discharge from the eyes** (opposite of *Euphrasia*).
- Discharge from the nose and eyes in copious amounts
- Nose eventually gets completely obstructed
- Frequently heaviness in the middle of the forehead and/or a headache that gets better when the nose drains freely
- Frequently begins on the **left side**
- Worse in the late afternoon and evening, and from being in a warm room
- Better from open air, cold air

Apis mellifica **(honeybee):** More times than not, this is the right remedy for allergic reactions to beestings. Be prepared to give it on the way to the emergency room. Use for any severe allergic reaction that involves the following combination of symptoms.
- Very significant swelling of the eyes. Sometimes the eyes are literally bloodshot from swelling
- Heat and burning sensation of the face and the eyes
- Craves cold applications and is much improved by them

Table 14.5 Hay Fever and Other Acute Allergies Comparison Chart

Remedy	Better	Worse	Emotional State
Allium	Open, cold air	Warm, stuffy room; late afternoon and evening	Has difficulty thinking
Apis	Cold applications	Heat	Irritable; needs to move
Arsenicum	Warm applications; warm room; warm drinks	Cold	Anxious; fearful of serious, incurable illness
Euphrasia	Lying down in bed at night; coffee	Morning	No data
Nux vomica	Waking up in the morning; open air; eating meals	Warm room	Irritable; oversensitive to all stimuli
Sabadilla	Heat; being in a warm room; warm drinks	Cold temperature; open air	Anxious; timid
Urtica urens	No modalities	Water; cool, moist air; touch	No data

Physical Problems	Signs Guiding Your Selection	Remedy to Compare With
Stuffy nose; heaviness at the base of the nose	Bland discharge from the eyes and irritating discharge from the nose	*Euphrasia; Arsenicum*
Significant redness, swelling, stinging (like from a bee sting) and pain	Allergic reactions to bee stings; allergic reactions with swelling and redness; skin hot to the touch; much improvement from ice-cold applications	*Urtica urens*
Mainly right-sided problems; irritating watery dripping from an obstructed nose	Irritating discharge from the nose; improvement from warmth	*Allium; Euphrasia; Sabadilla*
Center of the problem is in the eyes	Irritated, itching, burning eyes; abundant tears; bland nasal discharge	*Allium*
Cold; prone to spasms	Stuffed, dry nose at night; sneezing and discharge from the nose in the morning	*Allium; Sabadilla*
No thirst; desire for hot food	Fits of sneezing that may sound like an automatic weapon; itchiness inside the nose and/or of the palate	*Arsenicum; Nux vomica*
Tendency to have hives and blotches	Allergic reactions to shellfish	*Apis*

***Arsenicum album* (oxide of arsenic):** Use when there is:
- Irritating watery discharge from the nose.
- Dripping from the nose, which is completely obstructed.
- **Burning in the eyes, nose, and throat, which gets better from hot drinks or hot applications.**
- **Right side is mainly affected.**
- Better from being in a warm room, warm drinks, and warm applications. (Compare to *Allium cepa*).
- Worse from anything cold.

***Euphrasia officinalis* (eyebright):** Always compare to *Allium cepa*.
- **Eyes feel irritated, burning and itching**
- **Tears are abundant and irritating, nasal discharge is bland** (exactly opposite to *Allium cepa*).
- Worse in the morning and from warm wind
- Better upon lying down in bed at night

***Sabadilla* (cevadilla seed):** The picture includes the following symptoms.
- **Remarkable fits of sneezing.** Some people sound like an automatic weapon
- Every fit of sneezing provokes tears
- Constant itching inside of the nose and/or the palate
- Worse from cold and open air
- Better from heat, being in a warm room, and warm drinks

***Urtica urens* (stinging nettle):** This remedy is specifically used for allergic reactions to shellfish. Look for:
- Itching hives with a prickling, burning sensation.
- Hives that look like red, raised blotches with white centers.

A Few More Conditions That May Require *Nux Vomica*

As you may recall from reading previous chapters, *Nux vomica* is often indicated for headaches, especially those that frequently come as a result of tension at work or working too much. The person who needs *Nux vomica* is very irritable during the headache. I can still remember the headaches I used to get from moonlighting in the emergency room after a full day of work and almost no sleep. *Nux vomica* 30C helped me quite a bit. It also helps people who lose sleep as a result of "working hard and *playing* hard."

Obviously, if you had spent the day on the trading floor of the stock exchange, and then went out with your friends and had a few drinks, and who knows what other "recreational" substances, your sleep would not be the greatest. The same idea applies to coming home from a large wedding party. An acute hangover may respond very nicely to *Nux vomica.*

Just remember, *Nux vomica,* or any other remedy, won't help a chronic alcoholic recover unless he or she wants to. One needs to see exactly what remedy is indicated, and that is a job for an experienced homeopath working in accord with other drug or alcohol treatment professionals. Nux vomica is just the King of all remedies, not just the King of recovering alcoholics.

And let's not forget about PMS, whose pain makes many women feel sad and irritable. This condition is terribly uncomfortable for the women who endure it month after month, but there's good news. Homeopathy can help and it's worth the attempt to gain relief. Sufferers really need to work with a trained homeopath that can help them make the right choice. There are many things about this condition that can complicate the selection process. Nobody wants PMS to continue!

Another important idea for you to appreciate is that homeopathy helps to cure all varieties of digestive problems. I certainly have seen many cases when homeopathic remedies provided significant relief for people with irritable bowel syndrome and even Crohn's disease. Treatment of these illnesses has to be provided by a trained homeopath. The famous label of "indigestion" covers so many various potentially serious chronic problems that advising you on self-treatment would be unwise.

When *Not* to Self-Medicate with *Nux Vomica*

There are times when it is best to seek the counsel of a professional homeopath.

- Always seek professional help for severe alcohol and drug withdrawal.
- Although a few recent clinical studies suggest that more complex allergic diseases like chronic allergies, asthma, and sinusitis can be successfully treated with homeopathy, to do so effectively you would almost certainly need the assistance of a trained homeopath.
- Recurrent complaints are more complicated to treat than nonchronic complaints, and thus these require the attention of a qualified homeopathic practitioner.

CHAPTER FIFTEEN

Helpful Hints Remedies for Common Ailments

"When the solution is simple, God is answering."
ALBERT EINSTEIN

My idea here is to offer you a homeopathic cheat sheet for acute conditions so you'll be able to orient yourself quickly when handling different types of situations, spanning from anger and kidney stones to sore throats and varicose veins. You may be able to get away just with using the information presented in this chapter, or you may need to return to a chapter that corresponds to one of the book's eight central remedies. Then, with the advantage of having a fairly good idea in mind of your remedy of choice, you'll swiftly be able to confirm its key symptoms or find out that you need a different remedy.

Please note: Some conditions listed in the following pages aren't included in the chapters on the eight remedies. In such cases, you'll be offered one or two choices of commonly indicated remedies for these ailments. When appropriate, I'll also talk about herbs and supplements that can be used to enhance the action of the homeopathy. Each description will include suggestions of an appropriate regimen for taking the remedy, herb, or supplement.

Remember, if you can clearly see the main characteristics of *any* of the remedies described in the earlier chapters, give that remedy *regardless* of the diagnosis and short recommendations you find in this chapter.

Allergies (Acute)
Also *see* "Hay Fever"

Take three 30C pellets of either of the following remedies every fifteen minutes three times in a row. Stop if there is a 50 percent improvement, even after the first dose. Stop if there is no improvement at all or if you feel worse. In cases of severe allergic reactions, take the remedy on your way to the emergency room.

Apis mellifica. This is for allergic reactions to beestings and for any allergic reaction with significant swelling, redness, and local pain. Often the victim also feels irritable.

Urtica urens. This is for allergic reactions to shellfish.

Herbal Preparations

A good addition to homeopathy is extract of eyebright and stinging nettles. (Herb Pharm makes a product called Eyebright/Nettle Compound; other herbal companies have similar products.) Take ten drops three times a day.

Anger

Chamomilla. This is for babies and toddlers, especially during teething, as well as for women during a difficult, painful delivery. Take three 30C pellets dry or in water each time there is an angry outburst. Stop if better. Also stop and consult a homeopath if there was no effect at all after the first dose.

Nux vomica. This is for intense, overworked, stressed-out, driven, career-oriented people as well as for angry people who work many hours in a row and are on edge, their nerves raw. Take three 30C pellets. You may repeat the dose three times every fifteen minutes if there was an initial response. Stop when 50 percent better. See homeopath if there was no effect after three doses.

Anxiety
Also *see* "Stage Fright"

Aconitum napellus. This is for severe restless panic, frequently accompanied by a fear of death.

Argentum nitricum. Restless, wants company, talks a lot.

Gelsemium sempervirens. Feels paralyzed from anxiety, wants to be left alone. Quiet, shy.

Bites

Ledum palustre. Consider this remedy first for insect bites (such as from a wasp, tick, or any large insect), as well as for animal and human bites. Take three 30C pellets three times, every fifteen minutes.

Carbolicum acidum. This is for severe allergic reactions to bee stings, insect bites, and animal bites; it's also useful for anaphylaxis. The victim has a dusky red face. The skin around the mouth and nose is pale. The victim also reports a choking feeling and frequently becomes lethargic, but, even so, may paradoxically develop an acute awareness of odors. In cases of allergic reactions, a person develops hives over the entire body.

Call 911 immediately or go to the ER if you see these symptoms develop. You can always give a remedy on your way to the ER. Give three 30C pellets every ten to fifteen minutes until improvement or the arrival of an ambulance.

Oxalicum acidum. This remedy works well for bites from poisonous snakes or spiders if the affected part becomes numb and cold to the touch and the victim also reports violent pains and begins to tremble. It's imperative to rush the victim to the nearest hospital! Give three 30C pellets every ten minutes on your way to the ER.

Bladder Infection

Recurrent infections should be treated by a homeopath (which should give you good results). You have a very small window of opportunity. Try your remedy of choice for a few hours. If you don't get at least 50 percent better, start conventional treatment right away. I always advise taking the best remedy you can pick and going to see a conventional physician. If the remedy kicks in and you feel better before filling a conventional prescription, great. If not, well, you have a prescription in hand ready to go to the pharmacy.

Take three 30C pellets of any remedy in the following list three times at intervals of roughly thirty minutes. After initial improvement, you can continue taking the remedy every two hours until the problem is gone. If there is no effect at all after the initial three doses (meaning within two to three hours), then start conventional treatment.

Cantharis. This is the most common remedy for acute urinary infections. Severe burning pain with urination is the main problem.

Nux vomica. The person has a feeling of fullness and constant urging, but urine is passed in small amounts with a sensation of incompleteness and a need to urinate again.

Petroselinum sativum. This is frequently indicated in children. Severe itching deep in the urethra is the key. Sudden urges cause sufferers to jump and have pain if they do not urinate immediately.

Pulsatilla nigricans. The person experiences paroxysmal pain and very strong urges and cannot hold the urine. Pain gets progressively worse with an attempt to hold back the urine.

Sarsaparilla. The person passes large amounts of urine with severe pain at the end of urination.

Bruises

Arnica montana. Take three 200C pellets immediately after injury and before bed the night the surgery took place. To prevent bruising and other complications after plastic surgery simply use SinEcch (from Alpine Pharmaceuticals). It is *Arnica* conveniently prepackaged in capsules and labeled with easy-to-follow instructions. You can find it on the internet and in some health food stores. Please remember that taking *Arnica* too frequently may cause increased bruising due to the proving effect. Only take it twice—then stop.

I also recommend using a combination of *Arnica* and *Hamamelis* ointments (gel, cream, or lotion) to be applied externally twice a day.

Warning: Never apply these ointments on cuts (surgical or otherwise).

Ledum palustre. This is for bruises at the site of a bite or a puncture wound, or for large bruises after fractures. The area feels cold to the touch. **Bruises get better from applications of ice.** Take three 30C pellets once a day until improved.

Sulphuricum acidum. This remedy is used in cases when large bruises don't go away after *Arnica*. **Pain improved by warm applications.** Take three 30C pellets once a day until improved.

Burns (Minor)

Please remember to seek professional help (go to the emergency room) in every single case of a serious burn or when burns seem to be minor but are extremely painful and begin to blister. You can take a remedy on your way to the ER.

At home, start by placing your extremity under running cold water for about fifteen minutes. Never place ice directly on your skin!

For minor burns only, aloe vera ointments (cream, lotions) are effective. Do not apply ointment in cases of blisters or broken skin.

Use remedies in 30C concentration. Take three pellets every fifteen to twenty minutes until you see marked improvement. Stop after three initial doses, if you don't feel better.

Apis mellifica. Skin is red, swollen, and painful. Pain is relieved only by ice-cold applications. (*Cantharis* has the same characteristics in cases of serious second-degree and third-degree burns).

Urtica urens. This is for scalding from boiling or hot water. There is an itching sensation that accompanies the usual burning pain.

Chickenpox

In most of the countries, this illness practically has been eliminated due to vaccination. But if somebody contracts it, homeopathy is helpful. Be aware, however, that in the beginning of the illness you might need the usual remedies for colds and flu.

Later in life, the virus that causes chicken pox can be reactivated in a condition known as *shingles*. See the "Herpes Zoster (Shingles)" section for homeopathic recommendations.

Antimonium crudum. Take three 30C pellets three times (morning, noon, and night) on the first day.

Colds

Oscillococcinum. This is a proprietary single remedy produced by Boiron. It should be used at the first sign of a cold or flu. Easy-to-follow instructions are printed on the package.

For a more sophisticated, individualized approach, refer back to Chapter 8.

Herbs and Supplements

You may use extracts of echinacea and astragalus. Take ten drops of each three times a day (morning, noon, and night) for up to seven days.

Vitamin C. This is for adults without any chronic health problems. Take 500 milligrams in a chewable tablet every hour until you reach a daily dose of 3,000 milligrams (usually six tablets altogether).

Colic

Chamomilla. The most commonly prescribed remedy for irritable children who want to be carried at all times. Give three 30C pellets once.

If there is no effect, refer back to Chapter 11 to select a better remedy.

Constipation

Nux vomica. For frequent, ineffective urges and the feeling of incompleteness after a bowel movement. Take three 12C pellets every day for a week.

If there's no effect, refer back to Chapter 14. And if your symptoms are not in that chapter, consult a homeopath.

Cough

During cold and flu season take *Oscillococcinum* at the onset of cough for one day (there are clear instructions on the package).

Herbs and Supplements

Take extract of echinacea for a dry cough. And take extract of echinacea along with extract of mullein for a wet cough. Take ten drops of each three times a day. Also take 2,000–3,000 milligrams a day of chewable vitamin C. Usually this combination takes care of mild cases of uncomplicated coughing. For an irritating dry cough, also drink mint tea or suck on lozenges containing mint (peppermint).

Croup

Croup has the potential to be a dangerous condition. So give your baby the best remedy you know on your way to the emergency room. Better safe than sorry.

For the two following remedies, it is appropriate to give a child three 30C pellets every fifteen to twenty minutes. Stop if there is a significant improvement, and then give an additional dose each time the child begins to feel worse. Discontinue if there is no effect after three repetitions. For more details, refer back to Chapter 8.

Aconitum napellus. This is for the very beginning of illness. The child is morbidly scared.

Spongia tosta. This is good for later in the course of the illness or at the onset if there was never an *Aconitum* stage. The child improves from warm drinks.

Detoxification from Drugs or Alcohol

Consider the following two remedies. For either, it is appropriate to take three 30C pellets three times a day (morning, noon, and night). Also refer back to Chapters 13 and 14.

Nux vomica. This remedy is the absolute king of detox. The person who needs it is usually extremely sensitive to all sensory stimulation and is irritable and angry.

Ignatia amara. Consider this remedy if there is a prominent hysterical, emotional component to the detoxification process with a lot of sighing and crying.

Diarrhea

For more details, refer back to Chapter 14. If the remedy you choose is correct, episodes will become less and less frequent. Take three 30C pellets after each episode of diarrhea.

Arsenicum album. This is for food poisoning and is the first consideration in any case of diarrhea.

Podophyllum. This is for explosive, noisy diarrhea that soils the toilet bowl and frequently also the buttocks. The sufferer feels very weak after each stool.

Veratrum album. This is for profuse, odorless stool that often looks like rice water. Simultaneously the person has forceful vomiting and becomes weak with cold sweat.

Additional Measures

It is all right to take over-the-counter medications that contain bismuth, such as Pepto-Bismol, as these don't interfere with homeopathy. And be sure to drink a lot of liquids containing sodium, potassium, and some type of sugar (for example, Gatorade). In addition, stop eating sugar, carbohydrates, dairy, and spicy food. If you cannot live on small quantities of food, consider the BRAT diet (banana, white rice, grated apple, and plain toast). I prefer a combination of rice and tea (black or green) without sugar.

Ear Infections (Acute)

Warning: Always go see a doctor if there is discharge from the ear.
See a clear description of major homeopathic remedies in Chapter 10.

Herbs

Put a few drops of lukewarm mullein oil in the ear to stop the pain. Do not infuse the ear in this way if there is discharge.

Fainting

Carbo vegetabilis. Take three 30C pellets every fifteen minutes until better, a maximum of three times. Stop taking it if there is no effect after these three doses.

Fatigue (Acute)

For more details, refer back to Chapter 12. Take three 30C pellets of one of the two following remedies three times a day for up to a week. Stop if there is significant improvement. Also discontinue if there is no improvement at all in three days.

China. Use after the loss of fluid (including prolonged bleeding).

Gelsemium sempervirens. This is frequently indicated after mononucleosis. Always think about this remedy in cases of fatigue that accompany neurological problems.

Fear of Dentists, Doctors, and Surgery

Aconitum napellus. This is for people who are morbidly scared with a fear of death. Also for fear that keeps people, including children, from going to a doctor or a dentist even in the case of an emergency. Take three 30C pellets the morning of the scheduled visit and immediately beforehand.

Fever

See the "Colds" section in this chapter and refer back to Chapter 10 for more details.

Flu

See the "Colds" section in this chapter and refer back to Chapter 8 for more details.

Food Poisoning

Arsenicum album. Take three 30C pellets every fifteen minutes three to five times. Stop if there is a significant improvement even after the first dose. Also discontinue if there is no improvement after the third dose.

Fractures

Aconitum napellus. If there is initial shock with severe fear, take three 200C or 30C pellets a few times at fifteen- to twenty-minute intervals. Stop if there is significant improvement. Also discontinue if there is no change after the first two doses.

Arnica montana. Give three 200C pellets within the first hours after the fracture. May be repeated if necessary. This remedy reduces bruising, swelling, and pain.

Bryonia alba. The person cannot even sneeze, as any movement causes severe, sharp pain. Give three 30C pellets every thirty minutes. Stop if there is significant improvement. Also discontinue if there is no change after the second dose.

Hypericum perforatum. This is for crushed fingertips and is also a specific remedy for a compound fracture, an injury when there is a break in the skin around a broken bone. Give three 30C pellets three times every fifteen minutes, and then give three 30C pellets once a day for three days.

Ruta graveolens. This is for injuries to the shin, kneecap, and elbow, places where the bone is close to the surface. It is also for chronic pain after a fracture is healed but gets worse in cold, damp weather. Take three 12C pellets every day for twenty days.

Symphytum officinale. This helps bone to grow quickly. Give only after the fracture has been set! Take three 12C pellets once a day for twenty days.

Frostbite

Of course frostbite is a rare occurrence in most of the world, except possibly among skiers. But in some colder places (like Alaska, Siberia, or regions high in the mountains) it happens relatively frequently.

Secale cornutum. Take three 30C pellets every fifteen minutes. Stop after three to five doses or earlier if there is a significant improvement. Discontinue if there is no effect after three doses. May be repeated as needed if symptoms that initially improved come back.

Gas/Bloating

Frequently a chronic problem, this condition requires a visit to a homeopath. Following are two remedies that can be helpful in acute situations. Also don't forget about activated charcoal, as it can provide temporary relief from bloating and doesn't interfere with homeopathy.

Take three 30C pellets of either remedy once, then wait for about an hour. If there is no effect at all, the remedy you selected was wrong. If the effect is incomplete, you may repeat the dose as needed. Discontinue after three doses, or stop earlier if your symptoms improve significantly.

Nux moschata. This is for terrible distension experienced immediately after eating that's accompanied by constipation and foul-smelling flatus. Though the mouth is dry, there is no thirst. The person craves spicy food, becomes drowsy, and may even faint.

Nux vomica. This is for distention from overindulgence in food, drinks, and drugs. Also for distention after significant stress. The person usually feels worse a few hours after eating.

Grief

Ignatia amara. This is the absolute leader in the area of grief. Take three 200C pellets immediately after a breakup or bad news. If you are the bearer of bad news, try to give the remedy fifteen to thirty minutes before telling the person about the situation. On the first day, it can be repeated two more times. Then use as needed.

For more details about other options, refer back to Chapter 13.

Growing Pains

Calcarea phosphorica. Give three 200C pellets once. Then, in two weeks, start giving the child five 6X tablets of *Calcarea phosphorica* cell salts twice a day. Use them for two to three months. This remedy helps to form strong bones and teeth, and reduces growing pain.

Hay Fever

For a clear description of a few helpful remedies, see the "Allergies" section of this chapter and refer back to Chapter 14.

Headache (Acute)

Iris versicolor. This is frequently indicated for classical migraine headaches that begin with visual aura and end with vomiting. It is also for blurry vision and sometimes even blindness during headache. Take three 30C pellets every fifteen minutes a maximum of three times. Stop if there is a significant improvement earlier.

For more details, refer back to Chapter 12.

Head Injury

Arnica montana. Take three 200C or 30C pellets three times on the day of the injury. Please also remember that head injuries with even a short loss of consciousness require a detailed medical workup. Take yourself (or the victim) to the doctor or ER even if you (or they) feel good. One of the main symptoms of *Arnica* is to believe you don't need help, remember?

Hemorrhoids

Aesculus. Take three 30C pellets a day for a few days. Stop the moment there is a significant improvement. Also discontinue if there is no marked improvement after three days. Combine with homeopathic hemorrhoid suppositories.

Nux vomica. This is for painful hemorrhoids in combination with constipation in overindulgent, irritable people. Follow the regimen described for *Aesculus.*

For more details, refer back to Chapter 14. Remember that chronic hemorrhoids require a visit to a homeopath.

Herpes Zoster (Shingles)

For chronic, recurrent cases see a homeopath. It is appropriate with the following three remedies to take three 30C pellets twice a day for three days. If there is no effect, or if you feel worse, discontinue.

Apis mellifica. This is for lesions on the face, especially on the left side.

Arsenicum album. This is for pain that is burning which is relieved by warm applications.

Ranunculus bulbosus. This is the remedy of choice for shingles on the left side of the chest.

Supplements

Lysine. Take 500 milligrams twice a day.

Vitamin C. Take 500 milligrams twice a day.

Hives (Acute)

Chronic hives require a visit to a homeopath.

Urtica urens. Take three 30C pellets three times a day (morning, noon, and night). Stop if the condition improves earlier. Discontinue if there is no effect after three doses.

Indigestion

Take three 30C pellets of either of the following remedies three times a day for one day. Stop if the condition improves earlier. Also discontinue if there is no effect after three doses.

Arsenicum album. This is for indigestion from eating too much fruit. The person is frequently anxious.

Nux vomica. This is for indigestion from overeating, along with irritability and constricting pains.

Injuries

Arnica montana. This remedy should be always considered first. Refer back to Chapter 9 for detailed information on the treatment of injuries.

Insect Bites and Stings

Give three 30C pellets of either of the following remedies three times at fifteen-minute intervals.

Apis mellifica. This is for stings by bees and other small insects. Typical symptoms: The site of the bite is hot to the touch, red, and swollen. The person is frequently (but not always) irritable.

Ledum palustre. For stings and bites by large insects (wasps, for example). The site of the bite is cold to the touch and has a bluish tinge in color. Paradoxically, the cold-to-the-touch lesion improves from exposure to extreme cold.

Insomnia (Temporary)

Coffea cruda. Take three 30C pellets once. If the remedy does not work or stops working in a while, see a homeopath.

Kidney Stones (Acute Pain While Passing the Stone)

In this section, we are talking only about acute pain that occurs while passing a kidney stone.

Warning: A kidney stone must pass relatively quickly. If the stone does not pass in twenty-four hours, you must see a urologist. Longstanding obstruction can cause permanent damage to your kidney. It is better to involve a urologist rather early. You don't have to wait for a day. Do what seems to be reasonably safe. I would go sooner myself.

Take three 30C pellets of either of the following remedies three times a day. Continue for two to three days. Homeopathy also can help resolve the general issue of producing stones, but that requires consultation with a professional homeopath.

Belladonna. This is for terrible sudden pain, usually on the right side. The face is flushed and red. Hands and feet are cold. The person is restless and much worse from the slightest jarring.

Berberis vulgaris. This is for sharp, shooting, or constricting pain that radiates in different directions. More frequently, the left kidney is involved.

Mastitis (Breast Infection)

In my experience, homeopathy helps this problem very well. But frequently it requires the involvement of a homeopath. If you have no access to a homeopath and have tried a remedy without any effect, go and see a conventional physician.

Phytolacca decandra. Very frequently (but far from always) this remedy solves the problem. Take three 30C pellets three times a day for a few days. Stop after significant improvement or if the problem gets worse. Also discontinue if there is no effect in three days.

Mental Fatigue/Exhaustion

Picricum acidum. For exhaustion after long studies, such as cramming for exams, or after other prolonged intellectual strain. Take three 30C pellets once a day for three days.

Milk Intolerance in Babies

Benign in the majority of cases, this symptom could be a part of a more serious problem, such as the result of birth injury or digestive problems. If the vomiting persists despite treatment for more than a few days, make sure to consult with a pediatrician. Projectile vomiting in a baby warrants an immediate visit to a doctor. Better safe than sorry.

Aethusa cynapium. Baby vomits milk in curds soon after the end of feeding. To prepare a mixture for your baby, place three 30C pellets in a teaspoon with a small amount of spring water, then crush them with another teaspoon placed on top. Give the mixture to the baby after each episode of vomiting. If the remedy is effective, you will see vomiting happen less and less frequently. Stop if there is no improvement in two to three days.

Motion Sickness (Seasickness)

There are two predominant remedies for this condition: *Cocculus* and *Tabacum*. Give three 30C pellets of either remedy, for a maximum of three times, at fifteen- to twenty-minute intervals. Remember, in cases of seasickness, you'll see people who need *Cocculus* down below and people who need *Tabacum* up on deck.

Cocculus indicus. The person feels worse from open air, better from lying on a side in a warm room.

Tabacum. The person turns pale (almost green) and feels much better from fresh air.

Nausea and Vomiting

Refer back to Chapter 14 for clear information.

Nightmares

Nightmares respond well to homeopathy, although you may need to get a homeopath involved. I've seen numerous cases when parents gave their children *Stramonium* with great success and all I had to do was approve their decision. Unfortunately, this remedy is becoming more and more commonly needed.

Stramonium. This is for severe nightmares. A combination of nightmares, fear of the dark, fear of dogs, stammering, and clingy behavior points to *Stramonium* with a high level of probability. A combination of nightmares with even one of these other symptoms could be a good enough sign it is needed. The child also may be violent.

Give three 30C pellets and wait. If the condition improves in a few weeks and then comes back in a month or more, repeat *Stramonium* by giving three 200C pellets. You still may need to repeat the dose every few months, but less and less frequently.

Pink Eye (Conjunctivitis)

This condition responds well to homeopathy. See a homeopath if the choice of the remedy is difficult or unsuccessful.

Give the remedy three 30C pellets three times a day (morning, noon, and night). The correct remedy improves the condition in twenty-four hours.

Argentum metallicum. The person wakes up and cannot open their eyes because their eyelids are glued shut by an enormous amount of pus. Most frequently indicated in adults.

Pulsatilla nigricans. The most frequently indicated remedy, especially in babies and older children. The eye is red. There is yellow-greenish thick discharge from the inner part of the eye. In cases of allergic inflammation of the eye, there is a tremendous itching.

Herbs

Wash the eyes (first the healthy eye and then the sick one) three to four times a day with either eyebright tea or eyebright extract that's been diluted 1:15 in distilled water.

Warning: Ensure that the liquid is at room temperature. If there is a lot of pus, adding calendula extract in the same proportion is a good idea.

Poison Ivy/Poison Oak

Poison Ivy Pills. This product, which is manufactured by Washington Homeopathic Products, contains *Rhus toxicodendron* 4X. The pills come with clear instructions for use. The company claims an 80 percent success rate and also advises customers to use the product for prevention. Most of my patients find it effective if it is started at the first sign of trouble.

Shingles
See "Herpes Zoster (Shingles)"

Sinusitis (Acute)

Treatment of sinusitis, both acute and chronic, is a definite forte of homeopathy. Best results are achieved when it is treated by an experienced homeopath. On the other hand, if you catch the first episode of sinusitis with the correct remedy, the problem may be solved for a long time.

Constitutional treatment may take longer than one appointment (just as it does for the treatment of any other type of illness). In cases of acute problems, just try your best. Remember, if you fail, antibiotics are always an option. After a course of antibiotics is completed, see a homeopath for constitutional treatment.

Take three 30C pellets of any of the following remedies three times a day for three days. Stop any time there is significant improvement. Discontinue after three days.

Hydrastis canadensis. This is indicated when nasal discharge is green, copious, and thick. There is significant postnasal drip, frequently along with a sore throat. People who need it usually are constipated.

Kali bichromicum. This remedy is indicated significantly more often than *Hydrastis*. Nasal discharge is gluey, sticky, thick greenish-yellow, and comes out in long strings. The voice sounds nasal due to complete nasal obstruction that often is present. There's a significant heaviness, fullness, and burning pain at the root of the nose. If there is any problem with the stools, it's usually diarrhea. (The *Hydrastis canadensis* picture has constipation.)

Mercurius vivus. This is also frequently indicated, but unlike cases of *Kali* and *Hydrastis,* the green nasal discharge flows easily and doesn't create long strings of mucous. It is most frequently indicated in cases of frontal sinusitis. Pains are worse at night. Offensive breath. Tooth imprints on a coated, dirty-looking tongue. Also drooling. You can easily appreciate this symptom if you see wet spots on the pillow in the morning.

Herbs, Supplements, and Other Supportive Measures

Frequently these actions alone resolve most of the mild sinusitis cases.

- Avoid dairy and wheat. This alone makes a significant difference for a number of patients. Many patients also find eating pickled ginger and wasabi mustard helpful. Obviously, they put the wasabi on something (for example, on pieces of vegetable sushi).
- Washing out your sinus cavities with a neti pot solves many sinus-related problems. A neti pot is a small container with a spout.
- Use a humidifier at night.
- Boil some potatoes with the skin on and inhale the steam for five minutes twice a day with your head over the pot and covered with a towel.
- Drink hot tea with lemon, honey, and one-eighth of a teaspoon of cayenne pepper.
- Use echinacea and goldenseal extract (sold in the same container by many companies). Take ten drops three times a day for up to seven days.

Sore Throat

See a clear, detailed description of what to do in Chapter 10.

Spinal Injury

Take three 30C pellets three times a day for two to three days. In cases of severe trauma, take three 200C pellets three times every fifteen minutes on your way to the ER.

Arnica montana. This is for acute strains of the back as a result of heavy lifting or whiplash. The person in an *Arnica* state usually minimizes the seriousness of injury. Bruised, sore feeling. No urine after spinal injury.

Hypericum perforatum. This is the most important remedy for spinal injuries, especially when pain shoots up the spine or there is an injury to the tailbone. It is the remedy of choice for severe headaches and pain after a spinal tap.

Rhus toxicodendron. This is for sprains of the lower back and neck. The person feels worse at the onset of motion but gets much better as slow motion continues. Sitting for a long time makes things worse. Motion and heat make things better. The person usually has difficulties staying still.

Sprains and Strains

Take three 30C pellets of any of the following remedies three times a day for two to three days. Discontinue after three days.

Arnica montana. This is for a sore, bruised feeling. It is frequently indicated for people who have exercised too much and too long after a long break or they just started exercising. The person won't let anyone touch the injured site and might say: "I'm OK, it'll go away soon." (Of course, don't hesitate to use it even if this symptom is absent.)

Bryonia alba. Think about this remedy first for ankle sprains and strains. The person cannot tolerate even the slightest motion and wants to stay still.

Rhus toxicodendron. This is the most frequently indicated remedy for sprains and strains. The person cannot stay still, and is annoyed by stiffness and pain. Stiffness is the main complaint. The condition gets worse on the first motion but improves as motion continues. It gets much better from heat and hot showers. You can also apply *Rhus toxicodendron* ointment twice a day.

Stage Fright

Look in the "Anxiety" section of this chapter for descriptions of *Argentum nitricum* and *Gelsemium*. Also refer back to Chapter 12.

Sunstroke

For details, refer back to Chapter 10.

Glonoine. This is the remedy of choice for most cases. Give three 30C pellets one time. Move the victim into the shade, apply cold, and provide liquids. In severe cases, call 911 right away.

Surgery

Refer back to Chapter 9 for a detailed explanation of helpful remedies.

Teething

Chamomilla. This is the remedy of choice. Refer back to Chapter 11 for more details.

Varicose and Spider Veins

Varicose veins can be complicated by inflammation (phlebitis) and/or clotting (thrombosis). In these cases, seek immediate professional help. In many uncomplicated cases, a homeopath can provide effective help. One remedy is most frequently indicated.

Hamamelis virginiana. This works for many uncomplicated cases of varicose and spider veins. Take three 12C pellets every day for four weeks, and then stop. May be repeated after a few weeks' break, if still needed. Also apply *Hamamelis* ointment twice a day.

Wrist Conditions

Ruta graveolens. This is a specific remedy for wrist and tendon problems. For severe conditions and acute trauma, take three 30C pellets three times a day for three days. For longstanding problems, take three 12C pellets once a day every day for a month.

CHAPTER SIXTEEN

Combination Remedies
An "Easy" Solution

"If there is more than one answer to a question, then there is no answer."
—UNKNOWN AUTHOR

Of all homeopathic products on the market, combination remedies are arguably the most popular. This is evident because they are so prominently displayed in the homeopathic sections of most health food stores. Definitely bestsellers, these products seem to offer a simple and straightforward solution: one medication for one diagnosis. We can find combination remedies for almost anything that ails us and our families, conditions ranging from teething and head colds to premenstrual syndrome and hemorrhoids. Combination remedies sold in stores are proprietary to their manufacturers, yet this chapter is *not* an advertisement for them.

It's not hard to grasp the concept involved in manufacturing combination remedies. Two or more remedies known to relieve a particular symptom are combined in the same tablet. The expectation is that either the chosen remedies will enhance each other's actions, or that at least one of the remedies will be exactly what the patient needs.

These remedies exist right on the border between conventional allopathic medicine and homeopathic medicine. On one hand, these preparations are used to provide temporary relief for the symptoms of minor ailments in the same way as conventional drugs: through suppression. On the other hand, the components of these combination remedies are homeopathically prepared substances. Their proponents argue that the remedies are much better than conventional drugs, as they have no side effects.

But although they can be effective, the combination remedies are prescribed for conditions and not for individuals. That's not classically homeopathic in principle. To pick one, you just need to read the label. It tells you "cough remedy" or "teething remedy" and you just go ahead and use it.

Ideally, you would want to visit a professional homeopath for assistance in selecting a remedy for your condition. Homeopaths treat the whole person. We base prescriptions on the indicators that make people *different* from one another, rather than the symptoms that make everyone the same.

What combination remedies do instead is to offer a quick fix to the public.

Pros and Cons of Combination Remedies

As all combination remedies are proprietary medications, I feel uncomfortable rating their efficacy. Nonetheless, I don't want to leave you guessing about them without reliable information. So, let me just say that, in my experience, all the major homeopathic manufacturers produce equally good combination preparations. I never use them myself, however some of my patients report that various brands produce more or less similar results. It is also my understanding that at the beginning of the twentieth century different companies sold and bought the recipes of efficacious combinations from each other.

This makes the process of selection easier. Major companies on the American market are Boiron (France), Heel (Germany), 1800HOMEOPATHY (USA), Standard (USA), and Washington Homeopathic Products (USA). There are quite a few smaller companies out there, too, and companies change hands from time to time, which is a great benefit to the consumer. Mergers or splits of these companies mean only one thing for you: a continuous exchange of experience leading to better products.

What are these remedies useful in treating? They can provide some relief for self-limiting conditions in people with Level 1 or Level 2 health. There are impressive remedies for vertigo, inflammation, teething, and hemorrhoids, for instance. The major homeopathic companies use combinations that have been tested for years and been shown effective, but to reiterate, only for the *temporary* relief of self-limiting conditions. Treating serious and or chronic conditions with combination remedies isn't a good idea. It's conceivable that a combination may harm someone weaker and more sensitive.

An important reason for caution when taking combination remedies is that they're examples of polypharmacy, the act of prescribing multiple medications instead of a single remedy at one time. Classical homeopaths say that the danger of prolonged use of these products is that they might cause confusion in the body. You should avoid combination remedies, or any other homeopathic preparations, while you are receiving professional homeopathic care, as these preparations might interfere with the progress of treatment. But, in my experience, the use of many popular combination remedies is harmless, as long as there is a clear understanding of what they can or cannot do.

One thing is certain: People like them. Frequently they do provide impressive results, similar to conventional medications. For many consumers, therefore, taking homeopathic combination remedies is a good place to start testing the homeopathic waters, so to speak. Combinations usually provide temporary relief of symptoms and require no thinking in their selection, whereas determining the *single* remedy that would interrupt a disease and stop it permanently requires due consideration.

The tradeoff is apparent: Single remedies require significantly more work on your part. Real healing requires an understanding of individual traits. Of course, if you want to begin with single remedies, the success you achieve will pay off big time. You can achieve a complete cure as opposed to the temporary suppression of symptoms.

ACKNOWLEDGMENTS

First, I'd like to acknowledge all my patients as my main inspiration. I learned so much from each of you and have been inspired by homeopathic cures of your medical issues, and for this I am very thankful. My family and friends have been another major source of inspiration and they also have been willing and supportive "guinea pigs" from the very beginning of my homeopathic path.

This book would never happen without an amazing help from Stephanie Gunning who has been an experienced doula for all my homeopathic books. For this book, she was an amazing editor and a patient partner.

I also would like to acknowledge amazing help by Megan Andrews, who helped with proofreading and managing various details of manuscript preparation.

As on all previous occasions, I would like to acknowledge my teachers who served as major inspirations for my homeopathic career. George Vithoulkas essentially revived homeopathy for our modern world and thought and inspired homeopaths everywhere. I was fortunate to study with him, too. Paul Herscu, Amy Rothenberg, and Roger Morrison thought me many invaluable lessons. Books and articles authored by these great homeopaths are at the foundation of all my homeopathic books including this one.

I also would like to express my deepest gratitude to the souls of my late parents, Emma and Boris.

END NOTES

Introduction

Epigraph. Sir William Osler (1849–1919). Source unknown.

M. de Voltaire was the nom de plume of François-Marie Arouet (1694–1798), a prolific writer. Source unknown.

Chapter 1: Is It Healthy to Be Sick?

Epigraph. The Chinese sage Confucius lived circa 551–479 BCE.
1. George Vithoulkas. *The Science of Homeopathy* (New York: Grove Press, 1980).
2. Rudyard Kipling. *The Jungle Book* (1894).
3. O. Henry. "Hygeia at the Solito" (1903).

Chapter 2: The Basic Principles of Homeopathy

Epigraph. Joseph Campbell. *A Joseph Campbell Companion: Reflections on the Art of Living,* selected and edited by Diane K. Osbon (New York: HarperCollins, 1991): p. 15.
1. Yellow jasmine, from the family *Gelsemiaceae,* is not to be confused with real yellow jasmine from Madeira. It's actually woodbine, not a true jasmine, from the family *Jasminum*.
2. Howard Gest. "The Discovery of Microorganisms by Robert Hooke and Antoni Van Leeuwenhoek, Fellows of the Royal Society," *Notes and Records of the Royal Society of London,* vol. 58, no. 2 (May 2004): pp.187–201.
3. Leo Spitzer. "The Etymology of the Term 'Syphilis,'" *Bulletin of the History of Medicine,* vol. 29, no. 3 (May–June 1955): pp. 269–73.

Chapter 3: How Remedies Are Made and Regulated

Epigraph. Aesop was a Greek fabulist and storyteller (c. 620–564 BCE).

1. Michael Quinn. "Homeopathic Pharmacy." In *Classical Homeopathy*, M. Carlson, editor. (Philadelphia, PA.: Churchill Livingstone, 2003): p. 150.
2. As you may have figured out already, the number in front of letter C multiplied by two will indicate the exact dilution of the remedy. For 12C, for example, 12 x 2 = 24 (dilution is 10^{24} times).
3. Avogadro's number (6.023×10^{23}) is the number of molecules contained in one mole of a substance. One molecule of a remedy substance in a mole is approximately equivalent to the 24X (12C) dilution level. In other words, mathematical calculations show that not one molecule of the original substance can be found in a homeopathic remedy at the 24X (12C) dilution level. This explanation is taken from J. Yasgur. *Yasgur's Homeopathic Dictionary and Holistic Health Reference*, fourth edition (Greensville, PA.: Vann Hoy, 1998): p. 25.

Chapter 4: Myths, Controversy, and Confusion

Epigraph. David McNeill. "Yoko Ono Sounds Off," *Japan Today* (February 7, 2009).

1. A placebo is an inactive substance, with no medication in it, used to control for psychological factors in clinical trials of medications; in studies of pills and liquids it looks, smells, and tastes just like the drug that's being tested.
2. A.G. Johnson, Surgery as Placebo," *Lancet*, vol. 344, no 8930 (1994): pp. 1140–42.

3. J. Kleijnen, P. Knipschild, and G. ter Riet. "Clinical Trials of Homoeopathy," *British Medical Journal*, vol. 302, no. 6772 (February 9, 1991): pp. 316–23.
4. K. Linde et al. "Are the Clinical Effects of Homeopathy Placebo Effects? A Meta-analysis of Placebo-controlled Trials," Lancet, vol 350, no. 9081 (September 20, 1997): pp. 834–43.
5. D. Eskinazi. "Homeopathy Re-revisited: Is Homeopathy Compatible with Biomedical Observations?" *Archives of Internal Medicine*, vol. 159, no. 17 (September 27, 1999): pp. 1981–7.
6. Benjamin Franklin. *Pennsylvania Gazette* (February 4, 1735).
7. National Center for Immunization and Respiratory Diseases. "Five Things You Should Know about COVID-19 Vaccines," Centers for Disease Control and Prevention (October 13, 2023).
8. W.B. Jonas. "Do Homeopathic Nosodes Protect Against Infection? An Experimental Test," *Alternative Therapies in Health and Medicine*, vol.5, no 5 (September 1999): pp. 211–19.
9. D. Castro and G.G. Nogueira. "Use of the Nosode Meningo-coccinum as a Preventive Against Meningitis," *Journal of American Institute of Homeopathy*, vol. 68 (1975): pp. 211–9.
10. Samuel Hahnemann. *Organon of the Medical Art*, translated by W.B. O'Reilly. (Palo Alto, CA.: Birdcage Press, 2001): paragraph 273.
11. E. Bach, as cited in J. Winston. *The Faces of Homeopathy* (Tawa, New Zealand: Great Auk Publishing, 1999): p. 187.

Chapter 5: Your Visit to the Homeopath

Epigraph. O. Henry (William Sidney Porter). "Jeff Peters as a Personal Magnet," *The Gentle Grafter* (1908).

Chapter 7: Stramonium

Epigraph. Author unknown; source: Romina Avila. "PTSD Quotes," HealthyPlace.com (accessed August 15, 2024).

Chapter 8: Aconitum

Epigraph. Aeschylus (524–456 BCE).
1. John Henry Clarke. *A Dictionary of Practical Materia Medica* (1900).
2. James Tyler Kent. *Lectures on Homeopathic Materia Medica* (1905).

Chapter 9: Arnica

Epigraph. Leonard Cohen. *The Favorite Game: A Novel* (New York: Vintage, 2003).
1. Samuel Hahnemann. *Materia Medica Pura, volume 1* [Original edition 1830] (New Delhi, India: B. Jain Publishers, 1996): p. 89.
2. *Hildegard's Healing Plants: From Her Medieval Classic Physica* (Boston, MA.: Beacon Press, 2002).
3. A modality is a condition that makes the ill person, or a particular symptom, better or worse. It is a circumstance giving rise to an increase or a decrease of a symptom. For instance, the patient is worse (<) from wet weather, after midnight, and from cold drinks. Or the patient is better (>) from heat, from elevating the head, and from warm or hot drinks. Source is *Yasgur's Homeopathic Dictionary* by J. Yasgur (Greenville, PA.: Van Hoy Publishers, 1998): p. 155.
4. R. Morrison with N. Herrick. "The Bali Tragedy—Homeopaths on Hand to Help," *Homeopathy Today* (December 2002).

Chapter 10: Belladonna

Epigraph. Daniel Boone. *Daniel Boone: His Own Story and The Adventures of Daniel Boone, Kentucky Rifleman* (Mineola, N.Y.: Dover, 2010). Originally published in the mid-1800s.

Chapter 11: Chamomilla

Epigraph. Beatrix Potter. *The Tale of Peter Rabbit* (1902).
1. Website: holistic-online.com/herbal-med/_herbs/h44.htm
2. Varro E. Tyler. *The New Honest Herbal, third edition* (New York: Pharmaceutical Products Press, 1993): p. 84.
3. M.L. Tyler. Homeopathic Drug Pictures (New Delhi, India: B. Jain Publishers, 1998): p. 236.
4. N.M. Choudhuri. *A Study on Materia Medica* (New Delhi, India: B. Jain Publishers, 2003): p. 270.

Chapter 12: Gelsemium

Epigraph. Eddie Albert (1906–2005). Source unknown.
1. Harvey Wickes Felter and John Uri Lloyd. *King's American Dispensatory* (1898).
2. Ibid.
3. E.C. Grant. "Food Allergies and Migraines," *Lancet,* vol. 1, no. 8123 (May 5, 1979): pp. 966–9. Also *see,* J. Monro, J. Brostoff, C. Carini, and K. Zilkha. "Food Allergy in Migraine: Study of Dietary Exclusion and RAST," *Lancet,* vol. 2, no. 8184 (July 5, 1980): pp. 1–4; and J. Egger, C.M. Carter, and J. Wilson, et al. "Is Migraine Food Allergy? A Double-Blind Controlled Trial of Oligoantigenic Diet Treatment," *Lancet,* vol. 2, no. 8355 (October 15, 1988): pp. 865–9.

4. B.K. Volger, M.H. Pittler, and E. Ernst. "Feverfew as a Preventive Treatment for Migraine: A Systemic Review," *Cephalagia,* vol. 18, no. 10 (December 1998): pp. 704–8. Also *see,* E.S. Johnson, N.P. Kadam, D.M. Hylands, a nd P.J. Hylands. "Efficacy of Feverfew as Prophylactic Treatment of Migraine," *British Medical Journal,* vol. 291, no. 6495 (August 31, 1985): pp. 569–73.

Chapter 13: Ignatia

Epigraph. William Shakespeare. *The Tragedy of Hamlet, Prince of Denmark,* act 3, scene 2. First Folio, 1623.
1. N.M. Choudhari. *A Study on Materia Medica* (New Delhi, India: B. Jain Publishers, 2001): p. 501.
2. Website: medical-dictionary.thefreedictionary.com/hysteria.
3. Andrew A. Monroe. Source unknown.
4. T.A. Hoover. "Opening the Home Medicine Chest—This Too Shall Pass . . .Homeopathic Help for Grief," *Homeopathy Today* (February, 2001).
5. You can see a photograph of Jack Lawyer and Seri the elephant in *Homeopathy Today* (October 2005): p. 23.
6. Dzifa Adjaye-Gbewonyo, Amanda E. Ng, and Lindsey I. Black. "Sleep Difficulties in Adults: United States, 2020," *National Center for Health Statistics Data Brief,* no. 436 (June 2022), U.S. Centers for Disease Control and Prevention.

Chapter 14: Nux Vomica

Epigraph. Vicki Baum (1888–1960). Source unknown.
1. N.M. Choudhari. *A Study on Materia Medica* (New Delhi, India: B. Jain Publishers, 2003): p. 733.
2. Samuel Hahnemann. *Materia Medica Pura* [original edition 1830] (New Delhi, India: B. Jain Publishers, 1993): p. 223.

3. Robin Murphy. *Homeopathic Remedy Guide* (Blacksburg, VA.: Hahnemann Academy of North America, 2000): p. 1249.
4. Vijai P. Sharma. "Characteristics of a 'Type A' Personality," mindpub.com (accessed February 26, 2024).
5. Elaine Woo. "Meyer Friedman; Doctor Identified 'Type A' Behavior," *Los Angeles Times* (May 6, 2001): p. B12.
6. Chris Bohjalian. *The Law of Similars* (New York: Vintage Press, 2000).
7. J. Jacobs, W.B. Jonas, M. Jimenez-Perez, and D. Crothers. "Homeopathy for Childhood Diarrhea: Combined Results and Meta-analysis from Three Randomized, Controlled Clinical Trials," *Pediatric Infectious Disease Journal,* vol. 22, no. 3 (March 2003): pp. 229–34.
8. Roger Morrison. *Desktop Guide to Keynotes and Confirmatory Symptoms* (Nevada City, CA.: Hahnemann Clinic Publishing, 1993): p. 305.
9. Website: Aaaai.org.

ABOUT THE AUTHOR

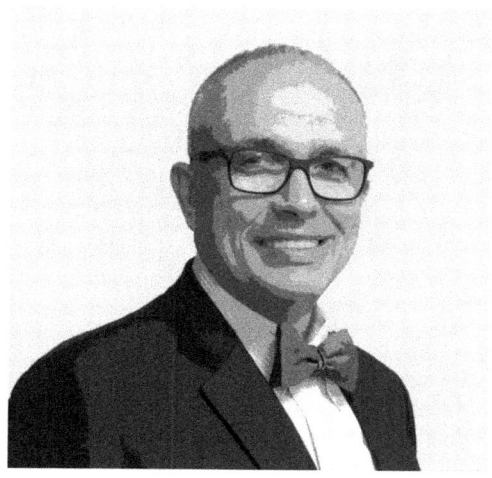

EDWARD SHALTS, M.D., D.HT., has been practicing homeopathy for over forty years. He has published two previous books and numerous articles on homeopathy and written chapters for several books. Dr. Shalts has also served on the boards of trustees of both the American Institute of Homeopathy and the National Center for Homeopathy.

www.ingramcontent.com/pod-product-compliance
Lightning Source LLC
Chambersburg PA
CBHW062112040426
42337CB00043B/3706